Cytotoxic Estrogens in Hormone Receptive Tumors

Based on the proceedings of a workshop on
The Use of Estrogens as Carriers of Cytotoxic Agents
in Hormone Receptive Tumors,
held at Diepenbeek, Belgium in September 1979.

Cytotoxic Estrogens in Hormone Receptive Tumors

Edited by

J. Raus

Dr. L. Willems-Instituut
Universitaire Campus
3610 Diepenbeek, Belgium

H. Martens

Limburgs Universitair Centrum
Universitaire Campus
3610 Diepenbeek, Belgium

G. Leclercq

Institut Jules Bordet
Rue Heger Bordet 1
1000 Brussels, Belgium

1980

Academic Press

A Subsidiary of Harcourt Brace Jovanovich, Publishers
London New York Toronto Sydney San Francisco

ACADEMIC PRESS INC. (LONDON) LTD.
24-28 Oval Road,
London NW1

United States Edition published by
ACADEMIC PRESS INC.
111 Fifth Avenue
New York, New York 10003

British Library Cataloguing in Publication Data
Cytotoxic estrogens in hormone receptive tumors.
1. Breast – Cancer   2. Breast – Diseases –
Chemotherapy   3. Estrogen – Therapeutic use
I. Raus, J   II. Martens, H   III. Leclercq, G
616.9'94'49   RC280.B8   80-40450
ISBN 0-12-583050-5

Printed in Great Britain by
John Wright & Sons Ltd at the Stonebridge Press, Bristol

PARTICIPANTS

Barel, A. Algemene en Biologische Scheikunde, Vrije Universiteit Brussel, Paardenstraat 65, 1640 Sint-Genesius-Rode, Belgium.

Benraad, T. Laboratorium Medische Biologie en Experimentele Endocrinologie, Katholieke Universiteit Nijmegen, Fakulteit der Geneeskunde, Geert Grooteplein Noord 21, Nijmegen, The Netherlands.

Blickenstaff, R. Veterans Administration Hospital, 1481 West 10th street, Indianapolis, IN 46202, U.S.A.

Bloomer, W. Harvard Medical School, Department of Radiation Therapy, 50 Binney Street, Boston, Massachusetts 02115, U.S.A.

Borgna, J. L. Institut National de la Santé et de la Recherche Médicale, Université de Montpellier, INSERM U 148, 60 Rue de Navacelles, 34 100 Montpellier, France.

Catane, R. Department of Clinical Oncology, Hadassah University Hospital, Jerusalem, Israel.

Cordi, A. Continental Pharma, Haachtsesteenweg 30, 1830 Machelen, Belgium.

De Boever, Vrouwenkliniek, Academisch Ziekenhuis, De Pintelaan 135, 9000 Gent, Belgium.

De Rijck, L. Limburgs Universitair Centrum, Departement WNF, Universitaire Campus, 3610 Diepenbeek, Belgium.

Devleeschouwer, N. Institut J. Bordet, Rue H. Bordet 1, 1000 Bruxelles, Belgium.

Edar, U. Schering AG, Müllerstrasse 170-178, Berlin 65, W. Germany.

Epsztein, R. Laboratoire de Chimie Organique Biologique, Université de Paris-Sud, Centre d'Orsay, Bât. 420, 91405 Orsay Cédex, France.

Formstechez, Laboratoire de Biochimie Structurale du Prof. Dautrevaux, Université de Lille, Faculté de Médecine, 1 place de Verdun, 59045 Lille-Cédex, France.

Forsgren, B. Aktiebolaget Leo, Research Laboratories, Biological Department, Fack, S-251 00 Helsingborg, Sweden.

Foster, A. Institute of Cancer Research, Royal Cancer Hospital, Chester Beatty Research Institute, Fulham Rd., London SW3 6JB, Great-Britain.

Fouquey, C. Département de Chimie Organique, Collège de France, 11 place Marcellin Berthelot, 75235 Paris-Cédex 05, France.

Gelan, J. Limburgs Universitair Centrum, Departement SBM, Universitaire Campus, 3610 Diepenbeek, Belgium.

Griffiths, K. Tenovus Institute for Cancer Research, The Welsh National School of Medecine, Heath Park, Cardiff CF4 4XX, Great-Britain.

Granitzer, M. Limburgs Universitair Centrum, Departement WNF, Universitaire Campus, 3610 Diepenbeek, Belgium.

Hamacher, H. Bundesgesundheitsamt, Institut für Arzneimittel, Postfach 330013, D-1000 Berlin 33, W.-Germany.

Harper, M. Tenovus Institute for Cancer Research, The Welsh National School of Medecine, Heath Park, Cardiff CF4 4XX, Great-Britain.

Heuson, J. Institut J. Bordet, Rue H. Bordet 1, 1000 Bruxelles, Belgium.

Heyns, W. Katholieke Universiteit Leuven, Rega-Instituut, Laboratorium der Experimentele Geneeskunde, Minderbroedersstraat 10, 3000 Leuven, Belgium.

Hochberg, R. The Roosevelt Hospital, 428 West 59 Street, New-York, N. Y. 10019, U.S.A.

Hoornaert, G. Katholieke Universiteit Leuven, afdeling Organische Scheikunde, Celestijnenlaan 200 F, 3030 Leuven, Belgium.

Hospital, M. Université de Bordeaux I, Faculté de Sciences, Laboratoire de Cristallographie et de Physique Cristalline, 351 Cours de la Libération 33405 Talence, France.

Ilsbroux, I. Limburgs Universitair Centrum, Departement SBM, Universitaire Campus, 3610 Diepenbeek, Belgium.

Janssens, J. Katholieke Universiteit Leuven, Afdeling Biochemie, Campus Gasthuisberg, B-3000 Leuven, Belgium.

Katzenellenbogen, J. University of Illinois at Urbana-Champaign, School of Chemical Sciences, 461 Roger Adams Laboratory Urbana, IL 61801, U.S.A.

Kelchtermans, M. Limburgs Universitair Centrum, Departement SBM, Universitaire Campus, B-3610 Diepenbeek, Belgium.

Kongsholm, H. H. Lundback & Co. A/S, Ottiliavej 7-9, DK-2500 Copenhagen-Valby, Danmark.

Könyves, I. Development Cancer Chemotherapeutics, Aktiebolaget Leo, Research Laboratories, S-251 00 Helsingborg, Sweden.

Lam, P. Manitoba Institute of Cell Biology, 700 Bannatyne Avenue, Winnipeg, Manitoba, Canada R3E OV9.

Lambrechts, J. Dr. L. Willems-Instituut vzw., Universitaire Campus, 3610 Diepenbeek, Belgium.

Laus, G. Vrije Universiteit Brussel, Pleinlaan 2, 1050 Brussel, Belgium.

Leclercq, G. Institut J. Bordet, Service de Médecine et d'Investigation Clinique, Rue H. Bordet 1, 1000 Bruxelles, Belgium.

Legros, N. Institut J. Bordet, Rue H. Bordet 1, 1000 Bruxelles, Belgium.

Lenaers, V. Université Catholique de Louvain, 73.20 Lab. de Pharmacie Galénique, Av. Em. Mounier 73, 1200 Bruxelles, Belgium.

Martens, H. Limburgs Universitair Centrum, Universitaire Campus, 3610 Diepenbeek, Belgium.

Mazaitis-Krijn, J. Radiopharmaceutical Chemistry, G. Washington University, Medical Center, Walter G. Ross Hall, 2300 Eye Street, N.W. Washington D.C. 20037, U.S.A.

Morgan, L. Department of Pharmacology, Louisiana State University Medical Center, School of Medicine in New Orleans, 2025 Gravier Street New Orleans, Louisiana 70112, U.S.A.

Mortelmans, C. Vrije Universiteit Brussel, Fakulteit Wetenschappen, Organische Chemie, Pleinlaan 2, 1050 Brussel, Belgium.

Mullens, J. Limburgs Universitair Centrum, Departement SBM, Universitaire Campus, 3610 Diepenbeek, Belgium.

Noel, G. Université Catholique de Louvain, Cliniques Universitaires, Service des Tumeurs et de Radiothérapie, Service de Biochémie, Av. Hippocrate 10, 1200 Bruxelles, Belgium.

Onkelinx, E. Limburgs Universitair Centrum, Departement SBM, Universitaire Campus, 3610 Diepenbeek, Belgium.

Paridaens, F. Institut J. Bordet, Rue H. Bordet 1, 1000 Bruxelles, Belgium.

Put, J. Limburgs Universitair Centrum, Departement SBM, Universitaire Campus, 3610 Diepenbeek, Belgium.

Raus, J. Dr. L. Willems-Instituut vzw., Universitaire Campus, 3610 Diepenbeek, Belgium.

Raynaud, J. P. Centre de Recherches Roussel-Uclaf, 111 Route de Noisy,

Romainville 93230, France.

Rousseau, J. Université Catholique de Louvain, Faculté de Médecine, Unité de Pathologie Générale, Av. Hippocrate 75, 1200 Bruxelles, Belgium.

Sandberg, A. Department of Genetics and Endocrinology, Division of Medecine, Roswell Park Memorial Institute, 666 Elm Street, Buffalo, New-York 14263, U.S.A.

Symes, E. Courtauld Institute of Biochemistry, The Middlesex Hospital Medical School, Mortimer Street, London W1P, Great-Britain.

Tait, B. I.C.I., Pharmaceutical Division, Mereside, Alderley Park, Macclesfield, Cheshire SK10 4TF, Great-Britain.

Tenenbaum, A. Institut J. Bordet, Rue H. Bordet 1, 1000 Bruxelles, Belgium.

Teuchy, H. Limburgs Universitair Centrum, Universitaire Campus, 3610 Diepenbeek, Belgium.

Töpert, M. Schering AG, Müllerstrasse 170-178, Berlin 65, W.-Germany.

Vanassche, F. Limburgs Universitair Centrum, Departement SBM, Universitaire Campus, 3610 Diepenbeek, Belgium.

Van Binst, G. Vrije Universiteit Brussel, Fakulteit Wetenschappen, Pleinlaan 2, 1050 Brussel, Belgium.

Vanduffel, L. Limburgs Universitair Centrum, Departement SBM Universitaire Campus, 3610 Diepenbeek, Belgium.

Van Lier, J. Centre Hospitalier Universitaire de Sherbrooke, Département de Médecine Nucléaire et Radiobiologie, Université de Sherbrooke, Sherbrooke, Québec, Canada J1H 5N4.

Vekemans, A. Institut J. Bordet, Rue H. Bordet 1, 1000 Bruxelles, Belgium.

Verhaegen, L. Limburgs Universitair Centrum, Universitaire Campus, 3610 Diepenbeek, Belgium.

Vereecken R. Katholieke Universiteit Leuven, St.-Rafaëlkliniek, dienst urologie, Capucijnenvoer 33, 3000 Leuven, Belgium.

Vervliet, G. Limburgs Universitair Centrum, Departement SBM, Universitaire Campus, 3610 Diepenbeek, Belgium.

Vilkas, M. Laboratoire de Chimie Organique Biologique, Université de Paris-Sud, Centre d'Orsay, Bât. 420, 91405 Orsay-Cédex, France.

Wittewrongel, C. Katholieke Universiteit Leuven, Campus Gasthuisberg, 3000 Leuven, Belgim.

Wittliff, J. Department of Biochemistry, University of Louisville, School of Medicine, Health Sciences Center, P.O. Box 3526, Louisville, Kentucky 40232, U.S.A.

Zeelen, F. Organic Chemistry R & D Laboratories I, Organon Scientific Development Group, Organon Int. B.V., P.O. Box 20, 5340 BH Oss, The Netherlands.

PREFACE

A major problem in cancer chemotherapy is the lack of specificity of most anti-tumor agents. These agents are very destructive to the dividing cells of the hematopoietic system and to the gastrointestinal tract as well as to the dividing tumor cells. The use of "pinocytotic" and "lysosomotropic" actions of cells has been proposed by De Duve as a measure to increase the therapeutic index of antitumor agents. Another approach of selective chemotherapy would be the use of hormone receptor transport mechanisms to concentrate the cytotoxic drug into receptor positive tumor cells.

A high proportion of human mammary cancers contain a measurable amount of estrogen receptors. The presence of estrogen receptors correlates well with the patients response to endocrine therapy but not with their response to chemotherapy. One can expect however that a receptor mediated chemotherapy will result in a more selective and efficient treatment of these receptor positive tumors. Several agents, containing an estrogenic and a cytotoxic moiety, have been synthesized in the past. It is not surprising that the affinity of these compounds for the estradiol receptor is very low since most of them were synthesized prior to our present knowledge of hormone receptor mechanisms.

It is extremely fortunate that prominent investigators involved in this topic have agreed to collaborate in a workshop to assess the gains made in this field of research, a field that has as major objective a more effective treatment of human mammary cancer.

In designing a cytotoxic compound that works through an estrogen

receptor mediated mechanism, the chemical reactivity of the cytotoxic moiety and the binding selectivity of the conjugated compound
have to be taken into account. To avoid cytotoxic effects before the
drug reaches the tumor cell, the chemical reactivity of the cytotoxic
moiety should not be too high and the drug should preferably be
activated within the target cell. The importance of binding selectivity
for obtaining a specific cytotoxic effect can easily be understood.

Three major problems are involved in selecting valuable cytotoxic
estrogens:
1) the limited amount of synthesized material available;
2) the need to screen a large number of materials for antineoplastic
   activity;
3) extrapolation of *in vitro* results to *in vivo* effects in the human.

These topics are discussed in considerable detail in this volume. It is
our hope that the book will help investigators in their efforts to develop improved drugs in the treatment of hormone receptive tumors.
We are grateful to the Nationaal Fonds voor Wetenschappelijk Onder-
zoek, the Ministerie van Nationale Opvoeding en Nederlandse Kul-
tuur, the Vlaamse Leergangen, Leo Aktiebolaget, Upjohn Company,
Searle and Co. and Cilag-Belgium for providing financial support and
to the staff of the Dr. L. Willems-Instituut, especially Mr. Tony Marx
and Mrs. Agnes Delsaer for their aid and cooperation in the production of this work.

The Editors.

CONTENTS

STRUCTURE-ACTIVITY RELATIONSHIPS OF ESTROGENS AND ANTIESTROGENS

OPTIMIZATION OF THE BINDING SELECTIVITY OF ESTROGENS

JOHN A. KATZENELLENBOGEN, DANIEL F. HEIMAN,
KATHRYN E. CARLSON, DONNA W. PAYNE, AND JOHN E. LLOYD

*School of Chemical Sciences, University of Illinois
Urbana, IL 61801, U.S.A.*

Introduction

Uses of Estrogenic Ligands: Hormonal Agents vs. Receptor Reagents

Estrogens and estrogen derivatives and analogs have been employed in medicine and biochemistry in a wide variety of ways, and, although the distinction may be somewhat arbitrary, it is instructive to differentiate between these applications, because the features required for the optimal activity and selectivity of an estrogen depend upon its intended use. The classical application of estrogens has been as hormones: modifications in structure and in formulation and dosage have sought to improve estrogen agonist activity, and hormone analogs with estrogen antagonizing activity (antiestrogens) were also developed. Regardless of the specific nature of the compounds involved, the goal has been to achieve a desired physiological or pharmacological effect that results from the hormonal action of the estrogen or antiestrogen. In such cases, the compound can be termed a "hormonal agent."

In contrast, for more recently developed applications of estrogens, the hormonal activity of the agent is often superfluous, while the specific affinity which an estrogen has for the estrogen receptor is employed for other purposes. As examples of such applications one might mention chemically reactive estrogens that can be used as affinity labeling agents to identify or characterize receptors (Katzenellenbogen, 1977 & 1978); estrogens attached to polymers for receptor purification by affinity chromatography (Bucourt *et al.*, 1978;

Sica *et al.*, 1973); tritium labeled estrogens to be used to assay the estrogen receptor content of breast tumor samples (Raynaud *et al.*, 1978); fluorescent estrogens for the study of binding kinetics (Dandliker *et al.*, 1978; Lee *et al.*, 1977); estrogen conjugates used in conjunction with fluorescent labeled antibodies for the histological classification of tumor samples (Lee, 1978; Pertschuk *et al.*, 1978), estrogens bearing gamma emitting radionuclides to be used as imaging agents for delineating the distribution of estrogen receptors in reproductive tissues and breast tumors by external gamma detectors (Katzenellenbogen *et al.*, 1980; Komai *et al.*, 1977), and finally, estrogens linked to cytotoxic drugs to be used as agents for the selective destruction of estrogen responsive tumor tissue. The unifying feature of these types of estrogens is that while interaction with the estrogen receptor is important, the major function of these compounds is not to elicit a hormonal response, but rather to convey a particular function or feature (chemical reactivity, immobilization, fluorescence, gamma-emission, cytotoxicity) to a particular site; the receptor serves to guide them to the desired sites in a selective fashion. To set them apart from estrogenic hormonal agents, such compounds can be termed receptorbased reagents, or more simply "receptor reagents".

Importance of Binding Selectivity

Estrogens have the capacity for interaction with many different sites. With both hormonal agents and receptor reagents, the desired binding target is the estrogen receptor. These are the specific, high affinity binding proteins found in target tissues and considered responsible for mediating the actions of estrogens. However, because estrogens are lipophilic, they can interact with many non-receptor sites as well.

Non-receptor binding can be divided into two categories, high affinity non-receptor binding, and low affinity non-receptor binding. The first category consists of complexation with high affinity binding proteins found in the serum, as exemplified by rat alpha-fetoprotein and human sex steroid binding protein. These sites are of high affinity (generally about 10-fold lower affinity than those of the estrogen receptor), and they demonstrate high structural and stereo-specificity in binding, although the profile of specificity is different from that of the receptor (vide infra).

The second category of non-receptor binding consists of low affinity sites, as are found on serum proteins such as albumin, as well as lipoidal phases (membranes). This type of binding is of very low affinity and is thus non-saturable over the usual concentration ranges utilized with both hormonal agents and receptor reagents. There is also little evidence of structural and stereo-specificity in this low affinity binding (although this may not be entirely true for serum albumin[1]), hence the common use of the term "non-specific" to describe binding of this type. (This term will be used throughout this paper with reference to the low-affinity, non-receptor binding.)

The relationship between the selectivity of action of a particular estrogenic agent or reagent and its "binding selectivity" (i.e., the ratio of its receptor to non-receptor binding) will depend upon its intended use. For example, with a hormonal agent, the binding to non-receptor sites may have no direct detrimental consequence other than lowering the potency of the drug; thus, structural modifications that reduce binding to serum proteins may be beneficial only in terms of increased potency.

On the other hand, non-receptor binding can be of greater consequence with some of the receptor reagents. For example, with fluorescent estrogens to be used as histological stains for receptor-containing cells, non-receptor binding could lead to an unacceptable elevation of background fluorescence. With labeled estrogens used to measure the estrogen receptor content of breast tumor samples, non-receptor binding can reduce the sensitivity of the assay procedure. In the use of affinity labeling reagents, interaction with non-receptor proteins can result in background labeling. However, in all these applications of receptor reagents under *in vitro* conditions, improvements in selectivity of the action of the reagent can be achieved by differential dissociation techniques *(vide infra)* or, in the last two instances, simply by purification of the receptor preparation to eliminate some of the non-receptor proteins with which the reagent is interacting. This is not the case with the applications of steroid reagents *in vivo*, such as with estrogen carriers of cytotoxic agents, where interaction with non-receptor proteins could lead to non-selective cytotoxicity.

Perhaps the application of estrogen receptor reagents that is most susceptible to the compromising action of non-receptor binding is the use of gamma-emitting estrogens as imaging agents for breast

---

[1] In preliminary studies (D. W. PAYNE and J. A. KATZENELLENBOGEN, Unpublished), we have found indications that the bis-phenolic, non-steroidal estrogens (e.g. hexestrol and diethylstilbestrol and their derivatives as opposed to steroidal estrogens) may bind to serum albumin more extensively than would be predicted from their lipophilicity (octanol-water partition coefficient).

tumors. In this case the reagents are used *in vivo,* and the totality of the non-receptor binding, both high and low affinity (as well as free reagent and metabolites that still bear the label), contributes to the background radiation above which the receptor-mediated uptake must be observable.

In conclusion, binding selectivity, that is the degree to which a particular ligand interacts with the desired sites as opposed to the undesired ones, can have important implications in terms of the successful use of estrogenic hormonal agents and receptor reagents. However, a full accounting of these implications requires a careful understanding of the particular way in which an estrogen is being used.

Binding Selectivity and Chemical Structure: Definition of an Index of Binding Selectivity, the "Merit Factor"

While the consequences of non-receptor binding may be different for different applications of hormonal estrogens and receptor reagents, it is useful to define an index of the binding selectivity of any agent. As binding selectivity will depend upon the structure of the compound, structural alterations can then be investigated for their effect upon this index.

We have defined the binding selectivity of an estrogen as the ratio of its receptor binding to its binding to the agregate of non-receptor binding sites.

$$\text{Binding Selectivity} = \frac{\text{Binding to the Estrogen Receptor}}{\text{Binding to all Non-Receptor Sites}}$$

We have mentioned that the non-receptor binding consists of high affinity binding to specific serum proteins as well as non-specific (low-affinity) binding. In the sections to follow, we will illustrate how the binding of an estrogen to the high affinity serum proteins can be minimized because the binding specificity of these proteins is different from that of the receptor. Thus, we can define a new quantity that is simply the ratio of receptor binding to non-specific binding. Because this ratio excludes the high affinity serum binding, we have chosen the term "merit factor" to distinguish it from the more inclusive ratio that was the definition of "binding selectivity".

$$\text{Merit Factor} = \frac{\text{Binding to the Estrogen Receptor}}{\text{Binding to Non-Specific Sites}} \tag{1}$$

In order to facilitate comparisons between estradiol and various analogs and derivatives, it is convenient to use measures of binding that are normalized to that of estradiol. The expression for the merit factor, therefore, becomes

$$\text{Merit Factor} = \frac{\text{RAC}}{\text{NSB}} \qquad \begin{array}{l} \text{RAC of estradiol} = 100 \\ \text{NSB of estradiol} = 1 \\ \text{MF of estradiol} = \dfrac{100}{1} = 100 \end{array} \qquad (2)$$

RAC is the ratio of association constants $(K_a^{\text{compound}}/K_a^{\text{estradiol}})$ for receptor binding and is generally expressed on a percent scale with estradiol being 100 by definition. It may be determined by direct measurement of the affinity of the compound and that of estradiol for receptor, if the compound is available in radiolabeled form, or it may be determined indirectly through competitive binding assay. NSB is the ratio of binding indices of the compound relative to that of estradiol for the non-specific sites, and by definition it is one for estradiol. It is preferable to use the binding index (nk) rather than the association constant (K_a) to characterize binding to the non-specific sites. These sites have such low affinity that they are essentially non-saturable; thus, only the product of the number of sites n and their affinity k (i.e., the binding index nk) can be determined.

Therefore, according to this normalized definition, estradiol has a merit factor of 100. Any other compound with a merit factor of 100 will have a binding selectivity that is the same as that of estradiol. Its affinity for receptor sites may be greater or less than that of estradiol, but its affinity for non-specific sites will be proportionately higher or lower, so that its distribution between receptor and non-specific sites will be the same as that of estradiol. Compounds with merit factors below 100 have lower binding selectivity than estradiol, and those above 100 have higher binding selectivity.

Relationship Between the Merit Factor, the Binding Distribution and the Ultimate Selectivity of Action of Estrogens

We will find that the merit factor concept is useful in studying the relationship between chemical structure and binding selectivity. However, we should not be deluded into thinking that such a simple ratio of affinities is totally adequate to express the distribution of a compound between receptor and non-receptor sites nor to describe the ultimate selectivity of its action.

First of all, in the definition of the merit factor we have excluded the high affinity serum binding, since it is assumed that steps can be taken to minimize the non-receptor binding due to this source (*vide infra*). However, in cases where binding to high affinity serum sites cannot be eliminated, the merit factor will give an overestimate of the binding selectivity of a compound.

Second, the merit factor is defined in terms of association constants; since high affinity sites will reach saturation as concentrations are increased while low affinity sites will not, the merit factor is a valid expression of the binding distribution of an agent only at concentrations below saturation of the highest affinity binding system. Fortunately, this will be the case for many applications, and even if high concentrations are used, the merit factor should still give some indication of the relative binding selectivities of different compounds.

Third, the merit factor is defined in terms of equilibrium binding indices and is thus an expression of the distribution of ligand under equilibrium conditions. There are situations in which receptor binding is being observed under "dissociating" conditions, that is, free ligand is being adsorbed or cleared. In such cases, the distribution of ligand will depend on the relative rates of its dissociation from different sites; generally, ligand will be preferentially retained by the high affinity sites, so the merit factor may underestimate the selectivity of the ligand distribution.

Finally, the merit factor is defined in terms of ligand bound to different sites. In applications such as tumor imaging, free ligand will contribute to the background, as will metabolites that contain the gamma-emitting label but no longer bind to receptor. In such cases, the merit factor may overestimate the selectivity of the distribution of radioactivity that is observed.

Nevertheless, despite its limitations, we believe that the merit factor of a compound is a very useful index of its binding selectivity, and that it is a particularly convenient basis for expressing how changes in chemical structures of estrogens affect the selectivity with which they may interact with biological systems. Depending upon the particular application in mind, one can determine what minimum merit factor provides adequate selectivity for the task, and above this level one can investigate chemical alterations that may provide beneficial contributions to the function of the agent.

Results and discussion

Measurements of Receptor Binding Affinity

There are numerous techniques that can be used to measure the binding affinity of an estrogen to the estrogen receptor when the compound is available in radiolabeled form with specific activity sufficiently high for its concentration to be determined accurately in the nanomolar range. Generally, receptor preparations that are cytosol fractions from estrogen target tissues, such as the uterus from immature rats, rabbits, or lambs, are used as sources of receptor. Binding determinations are usually made over a range of concentrations that span by an order of magnitude the K_d of the compound for receptor; in addition, binding measurements are made simultaneously over a range of much higher ligand concentrations (generally by the addition of a 100-fold excess of unlabeled compound or estradiol) in order that correction can be made for the contribution of low-affinity or "non-specific" binding.

Because the rate of dissociation of high affinity ligands from the estrogen receptor is very slow (especially at $0°C$), most techniques for measuring receptor binding involve removal of free ligand by adsorption, filtration, or washing. These non-equilibrium procedures effect a "differential dissociation" of ligand, that is, most of the ligand in the low-affinity sites dissociates, while dissociation of receptor-bound ligand is minimal. This increases the sensitivity of the measurement of receptor binding. The "specific" binding (which is the difference between total binding, measured with the labeled ligand alone, and "non-specific" binding, measured in the presence of a 100-fold excess of unlabeled compound) is usually displayed in terms of a Scatchard plot (Scatchard, 1949) in order to facilitate calculation of the equilibrium association constant. (Examples of such binding assays will be seen in Fig. 2) In such a plot, irregularities in the binding isotherm that might be indicative of cooperativity or of sites of medium affinity are readily apparent.

When the compound is not available in radiolabeled form, its binding affinity for receptor can be estimated indirectly through competitive binding assays. As these are generally run, increasing concentrations of the non-radiolabeled test compound are added to a series of incubations containing receptor and a fixed concentration of tritiated estradiol (which is just sufficient to saturate the receptor). The concentration range over which the compound competes with tritiated estradiol for binding to the receptor can be used to estimate its affinity for receptor relative to that of estradiol. (Examples of such assays will be seen later in Figs. 1 and 2) In addition to its applicability to compounds that are not radiolabeled, the advantage of this method is that it gives directly the ratio of association constants (RAC) that is needed for the numerator of the merit factor expression.

While binding techniques utilizing differential dissociation can be used to improve the precision of the measurement of bound ligand, an accurate determination of binding affinity requires a simultaneous determination of the concentration of ligand that is free. As generally applied, the procedures utilized for measuring receptor binding are quite deficient in this regard, as non-receptor binding can cause considerable error in the measurement of free ligand. Generally, the free ligand is considered to be the difference between the concentration of ligand added to the incubation mixture and the amount that is recovered as bound. However, if the bound ligand was determined by a non-equilibrium technique, which allowed differential dissociation of the labeled ligand from the low affinity sites, then this method will overestimate the concentration of free ligand and as a consequence, it will underestimate the affinity of the ligand, for receptor.

When the ligand is available in radiolabeled form and binding measurements are being made directly, these problems can be handled satisfactorily (Blondeau *et al.,* 1975 & 1978; Richard-Foy *et al.,* 1978). In such cases, the interaction with the low-affinity, non-receptor binding sites is determined directly in a separate experiment under equilibrium conditions (e.g., by equilibrium dialysis), and this information is used to calculate the true concentration of free ligand. The situation becomes more serious, however, when receptor affinities are being measured by competitive binding methods on non-radiolabeled compounds. In such cases, it is not possible to make a direct determination of the extent of low affinity binding by an equilibrium method on the unlabeled compound, because one cannot utilize radiotracer technology.

We have encountered situations where the contribution of low-affinity binding can cause a several-fold underestimation of the affinity of a compound. This can be exemplified with the compound o-azidohexestrol (o-N_3-Hex), a photosensitive estrogen thas has been used as a photoaffinity label for the lamb uterine estrogen receptor (Katzenellenbogen *et al.,* 1977). As we have reported, this compound binds extensively to non-receptor proteins (Katzenellenbogen *et al.,* 1977). Fig. 1 shows the competitive binding curves for this compound in lamb uterine cytosol before and after partial purification of the receptor preparation by ammonium sulfate precipitation (which removes the bulk of the non-specific binding proteins). It can be seen that the apparent affinity of o-azidohexestrol relative to estradiol increases by a factor of 6 with the purified receptor preparation.

There are other approaches to minimizing the discrepancies in receptor affinity determinations that are due to low affinity binding. In addition to purification as illustrated in Fig. 1, receptor preparations

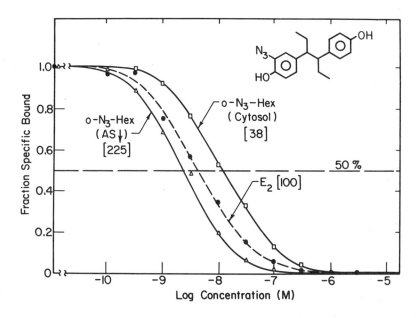

Fig. 1: Competitive binding assay of o-azidohexestrol (o-N$_3$-Hex) in lamb uterine cytosol directly or after partial purification by ammonium sulfate precipitation. The assay was performed as described in Katzenellenbogen *et al.* (1973). The concentration of estrogen receptors in the incubations was 2.1 nM, and ammonium sulfate precipitation was performed as described in Carlson *et al.* (1977).

that are as dilute as possible can be used; competitive binding assays can be run simultaneously with and without the deliberate addition of a non-specific binding protein, as will be described later. Finally, the addition of a small amount of an organic solvent can reduce the effects of non-specific binding dramatically. An example of such an experiment is shown in Fig. 2 with 1-fluorohexestrol (1-F-Hex), a compound we have prepared as a potential gamma-emitting breast tumor imaging agent (Goswami *et al.* 1980).

In the absence of the organic solvent, binding affinity determinations of this compound and estradiol by competitive and direct methods are shown in Fig. 2A and 2B. By these two methods the fluorinated hexestrol shows an affinity 19% and 29% that of estradiol, respectively. The addition of 7% dimethylformamide (DMF) changes these results dramatically: the affinity determinations of 1-fluorohexestrol increase 5-7 fold. The solvent has little effect on the affinity of estradiol (It decreases by 20%.), but in a separate equilibrium dialysis experiment (data not shown), it was determined that 7% dimethylformamide caused a dramatic decrease in the non-specific binding of

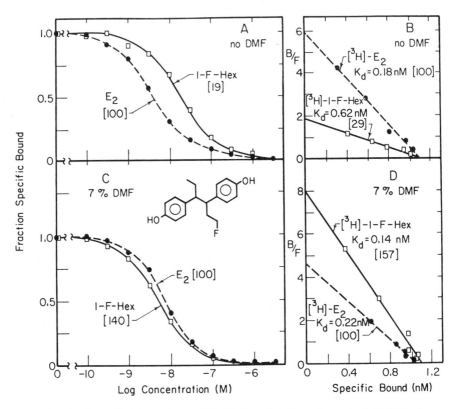

Fig. 2: Binding affinities of estradiol (E$_2$) and 1-fluorohexestrol (1-F-Hex) in lamb uterine cytosol in the absence (A and B) and presence (C and D) of 7% dimethylformamide (DMF). Competitive binding assays (Panels A and C) were performed using 10 nM ^{3}H-estradiol and the compounds in non-radiolabeled form, as described in Katzenellenbogen *et al.* (1973); (except that dimethylformamide was omitted from the experiments in Panel A). The concentration of estrogen receptors was 1.9 nM in these incubations. The fraction specific bound was determined by subtracting the level of residual (non-specific) binding evident at concentrations above 10^{-6}M and normalizing. Scatchard plots (Panels B and D) were determined in the same cytosol samples using the compounds in tritiated form. Specific binding is considered to be the difference between binding measured with the tritiated compound alone and binding measured in the presence of a 100-fold excess of unlabeled estradiol.

the 1-fluorohexestrol. Thus, competitive binding assays on lipophilic compounds that are run in the presence of low concentrations of an organic solvent can give more accurate measurement of their receptor binding affinity.

Measurement of High Affinity, Non-Receptor Binding (Serum Binding)

As was mentioned in the Introduction, estrogens can bind to high affinity, non-receptor binding sites in serum. Binding to these high affinity sites can often be measured by the same techniques used for the estrogen receptor, although in some cases dissociation rates are sufficiently rapid that some of the non-equilibrium methods cannot be used (Payne *et al.*, 1979).

We have done a thorough study of the binding of estrogens to the high affinity fetal rat serum binder alpha-fetoprotein (Payne *et al.*, 1979). This protein can be obtained in quantity from rat amnionic fluid, and is present in the serum of neonates, decreasing in concentration so as to be negligible at the time of puberty (20-25 days). Although the rate of estradiol dissociation from alpha-fetoprotein is too rapid to permit binding analysis by charcoal-dextran adsorption, hydroxyapatite batch procedures can be used. We have also measured binding to alpha-fetoprotein under equilibrium conditions by a miniaturized version of the Sephadex G-25 partitioning assay (Perlman *et al.*, 1969). Using this technique in a competitive mode, we have measured the relative binding affinity of a large number of estrogens to rat alpha-fetoprotein. A summary of the binding data is shown in Table 1, which also shows binding data from the estrogen receptor.

It is apparent that alpha-fetoprotein binds estrogens with high structural and stereo-specificity, but that this specificity is different from that of the estrogen receptor. For example, while the receptor binds the non-steroidal estrogens diethylstilbestrol and hexestrol with high affinity, they are bound very poorly by alpha-fetoprotein. The antiestrogen CI-628 and the fungal estrogen derivative zear-alanol are not detectably bound by alpha-fetoprotein. Conversely, while the receptor has lower affinity for estrone derivatives as compared to derivatives of estradiol, the reverse is true for alpha-fetoprotein. In particular, the photosensitive estrone derivative 16-diazoestrone, that has an affinity for the receptor only 0.5% that of estradiol, is bound by alpha-fetoprotein 131% as well as estradiol.

The major point to be made about high affinity, non-receptor binding is simply this: In terms of the preparation of hormonal estrogens and receptor reagents, it should be possible to design away from the high affinity non-receptor sites, because they demonstrate binding that is specific, but *different* from that of the receptor. Therefore, by the use of ligands such as non-steroidal estrogens that are bound well by receptor and poorly by the high affinity serum binders, or by inclusion of groups that interfere with binding to

TABLE I

Comparison of the Binding Specificities of Rat
Alpha-fetoprotein and Uterine Estrogen Receptor

Compound	Ratio of Association Constants x 100[a]	
	AFP[b]	ER[c]
17β-Estradiol	100	100
6-oxo-	1.1	21
$\Delta^{9\ (11)}$ -12-oxo	0.7	10
17α-ethynyl	3.0	191
17α (epimer)	0.3	10
Estrone	212	12
16-diazo	121	0.8
Estriol	1.6	5
Diethylstilbesterol	1.4	300
Hexestrol	0.2	300
CI-628	< 0.03	3.3
Zearalanol (P-1496)	< 0.03	32

[a] Ratio of association constants x 100 is $K_a^{compound}/K_a^{estradiol}$ x 100 :
Data are from Payne et al., 1979.

[b] Analysis on rat amniotic fluid (AFP) by the micro-Sephadex assay (Payne et al., 1979). Values expressed relative to 17β-estradiol = 100%, mean of 1-3 assays.

[c] Analysis on uterine cytosol receptor (ER) from immature or lactating rats or lamb y a charcoal-dextran adsorption assay. Values relative to 17β-estradiol = 100%, mean of 1-3 assays.

serum proteins but not with receptor binding, such as the 11β-methoxy group or the 17α-ethynyl group (Raynaud et al., 1978), one should be able to effectively eliminate the high affinity, non-receptor binding proteins as serious contenders for the ligand, and thus to improve the binding selectivity of the hormonal agent or receptor reagent.

If this strategy fails, it should still be possible to minimize this type of binding by using displacing agents. These would be compounds that are high affinity ligands for the serum binder, but bind to receptor only weakly. Their addition should displace the estrogen from the non-receptor site without affecting its binding to receptor. An example of such a strategy is to use androgens to displace estrogen agents from human sex steroid binding protein (Hähnel et al., 1979).

Measurement of Non-Specific Binding

Binding to low affinity, non-receptor sites (non-specific binding) can be measured only by methods that operate under equilibrium conditions, because ligand dissociation rates from these sites are very rapid. Also, because the sites are of low affinity, they are essentially non-saturable; so binding measurements can determine only the binding index, which is the product of the affinity and the site concentration, rather than provide estimates of affinity and site concentrations separately. Since the low affinity sites are not readily saturable, it is also not practicable to determine the affinity of non-radiolabeled compounds by competitive binding assays. The low affinity binding sites do not display much stereospecificity; in fact, binding to these sites has many of the features of a partition process, being non-saturable, non-stereospecific, and dependent mainly on the lipophilicity of the compound.

The correlation between lipophilicity and low affinity binding to serum proteins has been of great importance to pharmacologists interested in quantitative structure-activity relationships; of particular relevance to the problem of estrogen binding selectivity is the work of Corwin Hansch that deals with the low affinity binding of neutral compounds to bovine serum albumin (Hansch *et al.*, 1965; Helmer *et al.*, 1968). As a measure of compound lipophilicity, HANSCH uses the octanol-water partition coefficient P, which has become a widely-accepted standard (Leo *et al.*, 1971). Hansch derived the following empirical relationship

$$\log \frac{1}{C} = 0.751 \log P + 2.301 \tag{3}$$

where C is the molar concentration needed to achieve a 1:1 complex with bovine serum albumin. Since $1/C$ is proportional to the association constant or binding index nk, this equation can be rewritten as

$$\log nk = 0.751 \log P + \text{constant} \tag{4}$$

or, by normalizing to the binding index of estradiol, as

$$\log NSB = 0.751 (\log P^X - \log P^{E_2}) \tag{5}$$

where P^X and P^{E_2} are the octanol-water partition coefficients of a compound and estradiol, respectively, and NSB is the relative non-specific binding index as defined earlier. According to this equation, a compound with an octanol-water partition coefficient ten times that of estradiol will also bind to serum albumin with 5.6-fold higher affinity.

Serum albumin is a good model for the non-specific binding that is encountered by steroids; so, if this or a similar relationship holds for estrogens in general, then one should be able to estimate the level of non-specific binding of a compound simply from its octanol-water partition coefficient. A correlation for steroids that we have determined, based both on literature values for nk and log P, and values we have measured ourselves, is shown in Fig. 3. The relationship

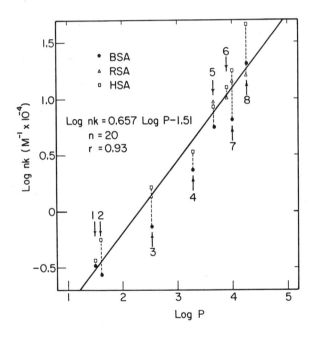

Fig. 3: Correlation between the binding indices (nk) of various steroids to serum albumin and their octanol-water partition coefficients (P). The binding indices are expressed as $M^{-1} \times 10^{-4}$. They were obtained from Westphal (1971) or determined in our laboratory by equilibrium dialysis or Sephadex G-25 partitioning (Perlman *et al.,* 1969). The values for P are measured (compounds 1, 3, 5, 6, 7, 8) or calculated according to Hansch's method (compounds 2, 4; see Appendix A). Three albumins are used: bovine (BSA), rat (RSA), and human (HSA). The compounds are identified by number: 1 - cortisone; 2 - cortisol; 3 - estriol; 4 - testosterone; 5 - estrone; 6 - progesterone; 7 - estradiol; 8 - diethylstilbestrol.

appears to hold very well for a variety of steroidal hormones over a considerable range of log P values; the sensitivity of nk to log P is slightly lower than Hansch found, however.

One complication with this approach is that for many estrogens of interest, the value of log P is quite large (in the range of 4-5). This makes the direct determination of the octanol-water partition coefficients difficult. There are two approaches that can be taken to circumvent this problem. First, the partitioning behavior of a compound in an octanol-water system should be related to its partitioning behavior in other systems. A convenient alternative is to measure the partitioning behavior of a compound by liquid chromatography in the reverse phase mode, utilizing a hydrocarbon bonded phase column and a mobile phase containing water with sufficient organic solvent modifier (methanol or acetonitrile) to provide convenient elution volumes (Carlson *et al.,* 1975; Mc Call, 1975; Mirrlees *et al.,* 1976; Unger *et al.,* 1978).

The second alternative is to calculate log P values. From the work of Hansch (1979) and Rekker (1978), it has become apparent that the partition coefficient of a molecule is an additive, constitutive property of the compound. Thus, one can determine the partition coefficient of new compounds by the summation of the contributions of its substituents or its constituent parts, using values that are determined empirically from model compounds. Hansch's (1979) method is a substitutive one and is particularly well suited for estimating the relative partition coefficients of a series of derivatives related by simple substitution. Rekker's (1978) method uses molecular fragments that are summed to construct the whole molecule. A brief explanation of the calculation of log P values of steroids is given in Appendix A. We have measured the chromatographic capacity factor k' (related to the distribution coefficient) of a large number of non-steroidal derivatives and have related these to their octanol-water partition coefficients calculated according to Hansch's and Rekker's method. All these correlations are excellent; an example is shown in Fig. 4.

There is another indirect approach to estimating the level of low affinity binding of a non-radiolabeled estrogen; this is to measure the perturbing effect that the addition of low affinity binders has on the estimate of receptor binding affinity in a competitive binding assay. We noted this phenomenon earlier in Fig. 1, when we showed that the apparent binding affinity of o-azidohexestrol was lowered when the competitive binding assay utilized unfractionated lamb uterine cytosol that had high levels of non-specific binding proteins. Clark (1974) has commented on the effect of low affinity binders on the

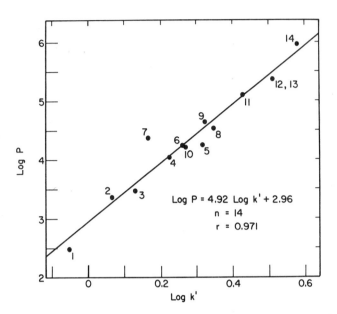

Fig. 4: Correlation between the octanol-water partition coefficient (P) and the capacity factor (k') of a series of non-steroidal estrogens. The log P values are calculated by Hansch's method (Appendix A). The k' values (Carlson *et al.*, 1975; McCall *et al.*, 1975; Mirrlees *et al.*, 1976; Unger *et al.*, 1978) are determined on a 4.6 mm x 25 cm C-6 reverse phase column (Laboratory Data Control) eluting with 70% methanol - 30% water, at a flow rate of 100 ml per hr on a Varian Model 4100 liquid chromatograph. Phenyltrimethylammonium chloride was used as the unretained standard. The compounds are identified by number: 1 - 1-hydroxyhexestrol; 2 - erythro-3,4-bis(4-hydroxyphenyl)-hexanoic acid methyl ester; 3 - 1-fluorohexestrol; 4 - 1-chlorohexestrol; 5 - hexestrol; 6 - 1-bromohexestrol; 7 - o-fluorohexestrol; 8 - o,o'-difluorohexestrol; 9 - 1-iodohexestrol; 10 - diethylstilbestrol; 11 - o-bromohexestrol; 12 - o-iodohexestrol; 13 - erythro-3,4-bis(4-hydroxyphenyl)hexanoic acid pentyl ester; 14 - 0,0'-dibromohexestrol.

apparent affinity of different estrogens to the receptor, and Levitzki (1975) and Zaagsma (1977) have discussed similar phenomena with ligands for the β-adrenergic receptor. While most of these earlier reports dealt with this issue qualitatively, we are currently working out methods by which such experiments can be used to determine quantitatively the non-specific binding index of an unlabeled compound.

The Merit Factors of Commen Estrogens

We have not, as yet, made a complete tabulation of the merit factors of all estrogens of interest. However, in Table 2, we have summarized the receptor binding affinity, the octanol-water coefficients, the non-specific binding, and the merit factors of several of the more common estrogens. The RAC values have been determined in our laboratory, or, where indicated, they have been taken from the literature. The log P values have been measured by us or calculated using Hansch's method (see Appendix A) and the NSB values were calculated from log P using equation 5.

Compared with estradiol, estrone has a lower merit factor; estriol, which has a receptor affinity less than that of estrone, has a larger merit factor because of its very low NSB. This effect is particularly evident with 6-oxoestradiol. The 11β-methoxy and 17α-ethynyl substituted estradiols have reasonably high merit factors. These derivatives are known to be highly selective estrogenic agents, but this is because these substitutions block their binding to high affinity serum proteins and retard metabolism (Raynaud *et al.*, 1973). The non-steroidal estrogens hexestrol and diethylstilbestrol have high merit factors; even though dimethylstilbestrol has lower NSB, its receptor affinity is so much lower that its merit factor is also low.

The Use of the Merit Factor as a Guide in the Design of Breast Tumor Imaging Agents

One class of estrogen receptor reagents that we have been particularly interested in developing are gamma-emitting estrogen analogs that will act as imaging agents for breast tumors that contain estrogen receptors (Goswami *et al.*, 1980; Heiman *et al.*, 1980; Katzenellenbogen *et al.*, 1975 & 1980). Such agents could provide valuable diagnostic information, as they would assist in tumor location. They could also delineate the pharmacodynamic features of estrogen-receptor interactions in the tumor, non-invasively and under *in vivo* conditions. Because the estrogen receptor content of human breast tumors is quite low (Mc Guire *et al.*, 1978), reagents with high specific activity are needed to assure that the receptor-mediated uptake of radioactivity by the tumor will be adequate for detection. In addition, as was noted in the Introduction, in an application such as tumor imaging with estrogen receptor reagents, the potential for the interference by non-receptor binding is particularly great. Therefore, in order to achieve satisfactory contrast between the tumor uptake and the background, such reagents will need to have very high binding selectivity (high merit factors). The results of earlier efforts to design breast tumor imaging agents have confirmed this requirement (Katzenellenbogen *et al.*, 1975; Komai *et al.*, 1977).

TABLE II

Receptor Binding Affinity, Non-Specific Binding, and
Merit Factors for Common Estrogens

Compound	Receptor Binding (RAC)[a]	Partition Coeff. (Log P)[a]	Non-Sp. Binding (NSB)[a]	Merit Factor (MP)[a]
17β-Estradiol	100[b]	3.97[c]	1.0[b]	100[b]
Estrone	12[c]	3.67[c]	0.60	20
Estriol	5[c]	2.54[c]	0.085	59
6-Oxo-Estradiol	20[c]	2.36[d]	0.062	323
11β-Methoxyestradiol	16[e]	3.30[d]	0.31	52
17α-Ethynylestradiol	160[e]	4.44[d]	2.3	70
Moxestrol[f]	40[e]	3.77[d]	0.71	56
Hexestrol	300[c]	4.24[c]	1.6	188
Diethylstilbestrol	300[c]	4.20[c]	1.5	200
Dimethylstilbestrol	20[c]	4.05[c]	0.87	23

[a] RAC = Ratio of association constants: $K_a^{compound}/K_a^{estradiol}$ x 100; by definition for estradiol RAC = 100.
Log P = Log_{10} of 1-octanol:water partition coefficient
NSB = Calculated relative to estradiol from Log P using equation 5
MF = RAC/NSB (See text for more detailed definitions.)
[b] Values by definition
[c] Determined experimentally in our laboratory
[d] Calculated by Hansch's method; see Appendix A.
[e] From Raynaud et al., 1973.
[f] 11β-Methoxy-17α-ethynyl estradiol-17β (R 2858).

In our initial attempt to prepare gamma-emitting breast tumor imaging agents, we synthesized o-iodohexestrol (Katzenellenbogen et al., 1975). While the corresponding o-substituted derivatives of steroidal estrogens are known to have relatively low receptor binding affinity, on the basis of our earlier work on estrogen photoaffinity, labeling reagents (Katzenellenbogen et al., 1973), we were quite certain that hexestrol bearing a single iodine, situated ortho to one of the hydroxyl groups, would still be bound to the receptor with high affinity. Indeed, this was the case, as this compound bound to the rat uterine estrogen receptor with an affinity ca. 40% that of estradiol (Katzenellenbogen et al., 1975). However, at the time, we did not consider the non-specific binding of this compound, and as it turned out, this compound is not useful as a receptor-based imaging agent because of the magnitude of its non-receptor binding. Using the methods described in this paper, we now calculate that o-iodo-hexestrol has a merit of only 1 (cf. Fig. 6). Furthermore, its binding selectivity is further compromised by what appears to be binding to some non-receptor sites of high affinity. While we did not characterize this binding in detail, it may be due to species that bind thyroxine, as protein-bound o-iodohexestrol and thyroxine co-migrate upon polyacrylamide gel electrophoresis, and the binding of o-iodohexestrol is in part displaceable by thyroxine (Katzenellenbogen *et al.*, 1975). A subsequent study of this compound by Komai *et al.*, (1977) confirmed our findings.

More recently, we have sought to develop tumor imaging agents more systematically and to examine homologous series of derivatives to determine what structural features convey optimal binding selectivity (Goswami *et al.*, 1980; Heiman *et al.*, 1980; Katzenellenbogen *et al.*, 1980). We have, thus far, concentrated our studies on analogs of the non-steroidal estrogens hexestrol and diethylstilbestrol. These non-steroidal estrogens have low affinities for the non-receptor serum binding proteins, and their chemistry tends to be less complicated than that of the steroidal estrogens.

Structure-Merit Factor Relationships in Three Series of Halogenated Estrogens

To date, we have prepared three series of halogenated estrogen derivatives: side chain halogenated hexestrols, aromatic ring halogenated estrogens, and α-iodo-α'-alkylstilbestrols. The syntheses of these compounds has been described in the literature (Allison *et al.*, 1980; Goswami *et al.*, 1980; Heiman *et al.*, 1980). Figs. 5-7 provide a graphical summary of the relationships between the structure of these reagents and their merit factors. In each figure, the receptor binding affinity, expressed as the ratio of association constants, is plotted with open triangles, the non-specific binding, determined from the calculated octanol-water partition coefficient, is shown as open squares, and their ratio, the merit factor, is represented by solid dots on the bold face line.

The side chain halogenated hexestrols (Fig. 5) show receptor binding affinities which are remarkably insensitive to the size of the halogen, decreasing from 130 for 1-fluorohexestrol only to 60 for 1-iodohexestrol. The relatively modest decrease in affinity is suggestive of two processes operating simultaneously that nearly offset each other, i.e. the somewhat greater tendency of the binding affinity to decrease as the steric bulk of the substituent increases (indicating the limits of steric tolerance at this site), and the somewhat smaller tendency of the binding affinity to increase as the lipophilicity of the substituent increases (indicating the preference

I-Halogenated Hexestrols

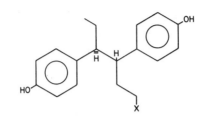

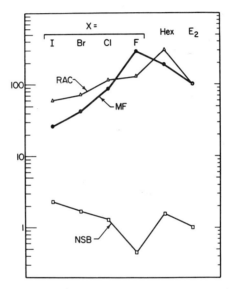

Fig. 5: Relationships between the receptor binding affinity (RAC), the non-specific binding (NSB) and the merit factor (MF) of a series of 1-halogenated hexestrols.

of this site on the receptor for non-polar groups). These opposing trends are almost in balance, with the result that there is only a small change in affinity as the halogen substituent is varied.

As the size of the halogen increases, however, there is a steday increase in the level of non-receptor binding predicted by the value of P. Therefore, the merit factor falls quite steeply with the increasing size of the halogen, decreasing from 250 for 1-fluorohexestrol to 26 for the iodo derivative. The merit factor of 1-flurorohexestrol is very high; it exceeds that calculated for the parent ligand hexestrol. Even 1-iodohexestrol may still be acceptable as an imaging agent, as its merit factor exceeds by a wide margin that of o-iodohexestrol.

The binding and merit factor relationships for the aromatic ring-substituted derivatives are shown in Fig. 6. In the ortho-substituted series, the receptor binding affinity is more sensitive to the steric size of the halogen than in the 1-substituted hexestrols. Receptor affinity in both the hexestrol and the estradiol systems is decreased to a comparable extent for the fluoro and bromo derivatives, but

ortho—Halogenated Estrogens

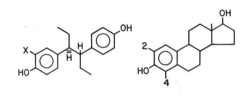

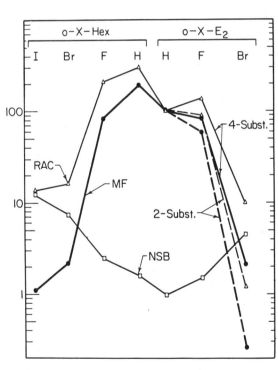

Fig. 6: Relationships between the receptor binding affinity (RAC), the non-specific binding (NSB) and the merit factor (MF) of a series of ortho halogenated hexestrols and estradiol derivatives.

hexestrol is much more successful in accommodating the iodo substituent. (Both iodoestradiols have RAC values below 0.1). We have previously suggested that the symmetry and conformational flexibility of the hexestrol ligand may account for the higher binding affinity of some substituted hexestrols as compared to the corresponding estradiol derivatives (Katzenellenbogen *et al.,* 1973). Because aromatic halogen substituents cause larger increases in lipophilicity than the aliphatic halogens, the merit factors of these derivatives are somewhat lower than those of the 1-substituted hexestrols (cf. Fig. 5), but they are still quite large for the fluorine-substituted analogs.

The structure-merit factor relationships of the α-iodo-α'-alkyl-stilbestrols are displayed graphically in Fig. 7. Receptor binding displays an intriguing trend as the size of the alkyl substituent increases. The hydrogen-substituted derivative binds with a very low affinity, but the binding affinity of the methyl and ethyl derivatives each increase by about a factor of 10, suggesting that the corresponding region in the receptor has a preference for a lipophilic group on the ligand. This region, however, does appear to have a restriction on the size of the substituent that it will tolerate, because the more lipophilic, but sterically larger n-propyl analog binds less well than the ethyl analog. This picture is consistent with the binding affinity of the isopropyl analog: the volume swept out by the isopropyl group is the same as that of the ethyl group, so it should be accommodated nearly as well. However, the isopropyl group is more lipophilic; therefore, this compound has the highest binding affinity of the group.

In this series, the level of non-specific binding also increases with the size of the alkyl substituent, but is does so less steeply than does the receptor binding. This suggests that the region of the receptor that accommodates the alkyl substituent has a greater preference for groups of high lipophilicity than do the non-specific binding sites.

As a consequence of these changes in receptor and non-specific binding, the merit factor increases quite sharply in the sequence hydrogen → methyl → ethyl → isopropyl, but it dips sharply when the alkyl group is propyl. The isopropyl analog with the highest merit factor in this series should have a binding selectivity comparable to that of 1-iodohexestrol and may prove to be a viable imaging agent for human breast tumors.

The Binding Selectivity of Halogenated Estrogens In Vitro

We have prepared four of the halogen substituted hexestrols,

α−Iodo−α'−Alkylstilbestrols

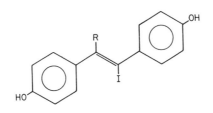

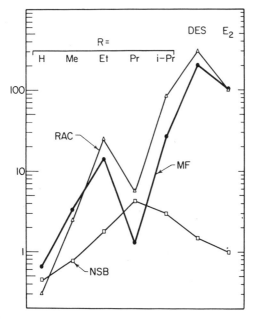

Fig. 7: Relationships between the receptor binding affinity (RAC), the non-specific binding (NSB) and the merit factor (MF) of a series of α-iodo-α'-alkyl-stilbestrols.

o-fluoro-, 1-fluoro-, 1-bromo-, and 1-iodohexestrol in tritium-labeled form with sufficiently high specific activity to do receptor binding studies. With these compounds, affinity for receptor measured directly by Scatchard analysis is comparable to that measured earlier by competitive binding assays.

Sedimentation through sucrose gradients is a classical method for characterizing estrogen receptor binding in cytosol preparations (Stancel *et al.*, 1975). The sedimentation profiles of ^{3}H-estradiol and the four tritiumlabeled halogenated hexestrols bound to rat uterine cytoplasmic receptor under low salt conditions are shown in Fig. 8. Under these conditions, the estrogen receptor runs as an aggregated species with a sedimentation coefficient of 8S. The specificity of the binding is confirmed by the displacing action of an excess of unlabeled estradiol (dashed lines).

^{3}H-o-fluorohexestrol and ^{3}H-1-fluorohexestrol have 8S peaks that appear comparable in size to that seen with ^{3}H-estradiol, while the 8S peaks seen with ^{3}H-1-bromohexestrol and ^{3}H-1-iodohexestrol appear to be much smaller. This is due to the lower specific activity of the latter two compounds (1.7 Ci per mmole) relative to the others

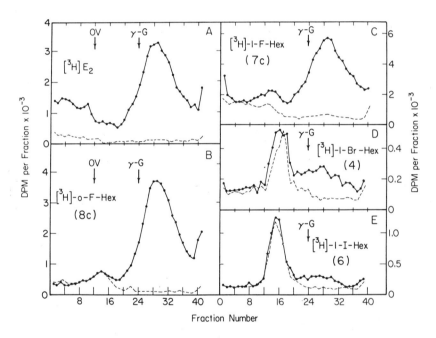

Fig. 8: Low-salt sucrose gradient analysis of the binding of estradiol (E$_2$) and four halogenated hexestrol derivatives in rat uterine cytosol. Formation, overlaying, centrifugation, and collection of the gradients was carried out according to Katzenellenbogen *et al.*, (1973). Sedimentation is from left to right. Gradients with the tritium-labeled compounds are shown as lines with points; gradients from samples incubated in the presence of a 100-fold excess of unlabeled estradiol to determine non-specific binding are shown as the dashed line. Carbon-14 labeled ovalbumin (OV, 3.5 S) and γ-globulin (γ-G 7.02) were included as sedimentation standards. In each case, the quantity of specific binding (represented by the area of the 8S peak minus the non-specific binding) corresponds to 0.61 - 0.84 pmoles of receptor per uterine equivalent.

(40-60 Ci per mmole); so the quantity of 8S binding in the last two gradients is, in fact, similar to that in the first three.

The major difference among these gradients is the size of the 4S peak. Binding in the 4S region of low salt sucrose gradients is generally associated with non-specific binding; this is confirmed by its persistence even in the presence of excess, unlabeled estradiol. The size of the 8S peak relative to the 4S peak is a direct measure of the binding selectivity of these agents. By this criterion, it is apparent that the two fluorohexestrols have binding selectivities that are quite comparable to that of estradiol, while the bromo and iodohexestrols have progressively lower selectivities. The ratio of the 8S to 4S binding of these four compounds and estradiol, together with their merit factors, is given in Table 3. The predictive value of the merit factor is quite evident.

TABLE III

Comparison of the Merit Factor and the Binding Selectivity
(Determined by Sucrose Gradient Analysis) of Halogenated Estrogens

Compound		Binding Selectivity[a] 8S/4S	Merit Factor
Estradiol	(E$_2$)	4.5 (100)	100
o-Fluorohexestrol	(o-F-Hex)	5.8 (129)	83
1-Fluorohexestrol	(1-F-Hex)	3.7 (82)	290
1-Bromohexestrol	(1-Br-Hex)	1.1 (24)	42
1-Iodohexestrol	(1-I-Hex)	0.62 (14)	26

[a] Calculated from the ratios of specific binding in the 8S region and non-specific binding in the 4S region of the gradient profiles in Fig. 8. Numbers in parenthesis are the 8S/4S ratios normalized to that of estradiol = 100.

The Binding of Halogenated Estrogens In Vivo: Tissue Distribution Studies

We have repeated the classical experiment of Jensen and Jacobson (1968) in order to investigate the tissue uptake selectivity of these compounds under *in vivo* conditions. Fig. 9 shows the concentration of radioactivity in various tissues 1 hr after intravenous injection of immature female rats with small amounts of ^{3}H-estradiol or one of the four tritium-labeled halogenated hexestrols. The tissue uptake (shown as vertical bars) is expressed as dpm per gram tissue and is normalized so that the uptake by the uterus is 100%; the absolute uptake can be ascertained from the data given in the figure legend.

There are a number of striking features about these data. First of all, the uptake by a target tissue such as the uterus is much more

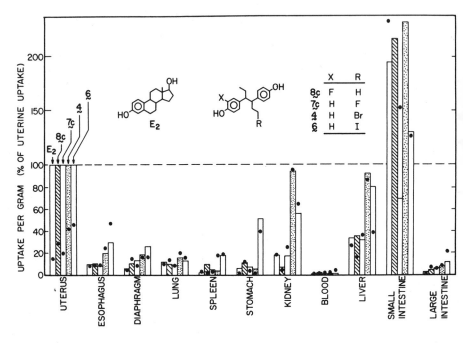

Fig. 9: Uptake of estradiol (E$_2$) and four halogenated hexestrols into tissues of immature (50 g.) female rats. Rats were injected intravenously (tail vein) with 0.3 μCi of the tritium-labeled compounds per gram of body weight in the absence (vertical bars) and presence (points) of an excess of unlabeled estradiol (to determine the non-specific uptake). After 1 hr, tissues were excised and radioactivity content determined by scintillation counting. Uptake levels are expressed as dpm per g tissue and are expressed relative to the uterine uptake (100%). The absolute uptake by the uterus (percent injected dose per gram tissue) was E$_2$ - 4.2; o-F-Hex - 2.9; 1-F-Hex - 4.2; 1-Br-Hex - 1.0; 1-I-Hex - 1.43. In experiments in which multiple (7-8) animals were used (o-F-Hex and 1-F-Hex), levels of both total and specific uptake were reproducible within 30%.

pronounced than that of the non-target tissues: esophagus, diaphragm, lung, spleen and stomach. Not surprisingly, some of the compounds show substantial levels in tissues involved in hormone metabolism (liver) and/or excretion (kidney and intestine). The labeled material which is extracted from these tissues consists almost exclusively of metabolites, while that from the uterus is essentially unmetabolized.

While the selectivity seen in the pattern of total uptake is attractive in itself, it is crucial to establish that the enhanced uptake noted in target tissue is due to receptor interaction, rather than to non-specific processes. In parallel experiments, the tissue uptake of these tritium-labeled compounds was determined in rats that were simultaneously treated with an amount of unlabeled estradiol sufficient to fully occupy estrogen receptors. In this case, the uptake into non-target tissues (level indicated by the dots) was essentially the same as before, while the uptake by the uterus was depressed nearly to the level seen in the non-target tissues.

Finally, it is most gratifying to find that the uptake selectivity of these compounds is successfully predicted by their merit factors. This is apparent in two ways: In the uterus, the non-specific uptake (dots) as a fraction of the total uptake decreases as the merit factor of the compound increases. The same trend is also evident in the uptake by the esophagus (both in the absence and the presence of excess unlabeled estradiol, since this is a non-target tissue), and the pattern is followed, to a large degree, by the other non-target tissues.

Finally, we have also examined the uptake selectivity of the two most promising compounds ^{3}H-o-fluorohexestrol and ^{3}H-1-fluoro-hexestrol in adult rats bearing DMBA-induced mammary tumors. As is seen in Fig. 10, the tissue uptake pattern of the two compounds in these rats parallels that seen in the immature animals. The uptake by the non-target tissues (esophagus, diaphragm, and lung) is approximately 20% of that of the uterus; this appears to be somewhat higher than was seen with these compounds in the immature animals (ca. 10%), but since mature rat uterus contains less estrogen receptor (ca. 10 pmoles per gram tissue) than immature uterus (ca. 30 pmole per gram tissue) (Tsai *et al.,* 1977), relatively higher non-target uptake is expected. Again, administration of an excess of unlabeled estradiol together with the labeled fluorohexestrol had little effect on the uptake in the non-target tissues, but it depressed the uterine uptake to the non-target tissue level.

Uptake by the mammary tumors is also shown in Fig. 10. In nearly every tumor, uptake of the tritiated fluorohexestrol is greater than that in the non-target tissues; this is particularly true with ^{3}H-1-fluorohexestrol (Fig. 10B). Excess estradiol also depresses tumor uptake to the non-target level. The receptor specific uptake in the tumors (the difference between the total uptake and the non-specific uptake) is about 25-30% that of the receptor specific uptake of the mature uterus. Again, this is consistent with the relative estrogen receptor content of the DMBA-induced rat mammary tumors (ca. 3 pmole per gram tissue) (Tsai *et al.,* 1977). It is noteworthy that the level of estrogen receptor found in DMBA-induced rat mammary

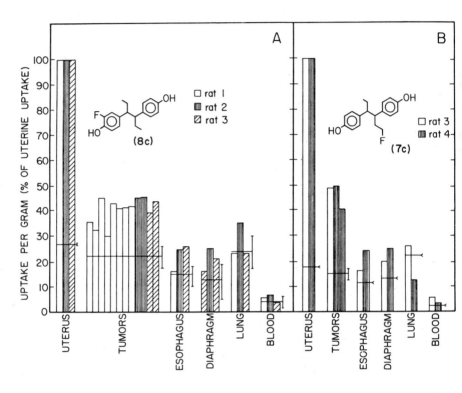

Fig. 10: Uptake op o-fluorohexestrol (o-F-Hex) and 1-fluorohexestrol (1-F-Hex) in adult rats (300 g) bearing dimethylbenzanthracene (DMBA) induced mammary tumors. The animals were injected and tissues were excised as described in the legend to Fig. 9. The rats had from 1 to 8 tumors per animal ranging in size from 0.05 - 8.7 g. The range or level of non-specific uptake (from animals pretreated with excess unlabeled estradiol) is represented by the symbols (⊢———⊣) or (⊢———<), respectively. The absolute uptake by the uterus (percent injected dose per gram tissue) was o-F-Hex (0.07-0.15) and 1-F-Hex (0.33-0.38).

tumors is in the same range as the median levels of estrogen receptor determined in human breast tumors.

Though they are preliminary, these *in vivo* tissus and tumor uptake studies suggest strongly that o-fluorohexestrol and 1-fluorohexestrol will be agents of sufficient selectivity to be useful as gamma-emitting imaging agents for human breast tumors. We are currently attempting to modify the syntheses of both of these compounds in such a way that they can be conveniently labeled with the positron-emitting isotope fluorine-18 (t $_{1/2}$) = 110 min).

Conclusion

In this report, we have tried to develop an understanding of the binding selectivity of estrogens. Careful analysis of the manner in which estrogens are used, as hormonal agents or as receptor reagents, has revealed that the consequences of non-receptor binding are dependent upon the actual use of the compound and the type of selectivity that is being sought. We have presented a careful explanation of the types of receptor and non-receptor interactions in which an estrogen can be involved and the ways in which these interactions can be measured, and we have proposed as an index of the binding selectivity, the ratio of receptor for non-specific binding, which we term the "merit factor". While the merit factor may be inadequate to describe binding distributions or selectivities in all situations, we believe it is a useful index to consider when structural modifications of estrogenic agents and reagents are being made in the hope of optimizing the selectivity of their action. A protocol by which the merit factor can be used in designing estrogens is presented in Scheme 1; it summarizes our approach to optimizing binding selectivity.

Scheme 1
Protocol for Using the Merit Factor in Designing
Estrogens With High Selectivity

1. Estimate the level of binding selectivity needed to achieve the desired level of biological or functional selectivity.
2. Choose a basic ligand structure that incorporates the needed function.
3. Synthesize the agent or reagent.
4. Measure receptor binding affinity (RAC) by competitive methods and estimate non-specific binding (NSB) from log P (measured directly estimated from the chromatographic k', or calculated).
5. Calculate the merit factor and compare it to the needed level of binding selectivity estimated in 1.
6. Consider structural modification that will increase RAC and/or decrease NSB to improve the merit factor.
7. Test the agents or reagents and examine how their merit factors correlate to the selectivity of their action.

Finally, as an example of the use of the merit factor in optimizing the selectivity of an estrogen receptor reagent, we have described our recent work on developing gamma-emitting estrogens as breast tumor imaging agents. In the studies we have carried out so far, it appears that the merit factor is an accurate predictor of the selectivity which these agents will display under *in vivo* conditions.

Acknowledgments

Support of this work through grants from the National Institutes of Health (AM 15556 and CA 25836) and the American Cancer Society (BC-223) is gratefully acknowledged. Fellowship support was provided by the National Institutes of Health (F32AM95718, to D. W. P.), by the Eastman Kodak and Proctor and Gamble companies (to D. F. H.), and by the Sloan and Dreyfus Foundations (to J. A. K.). The iodinated stilbestrols were prepared by Kenneth J. Allison, and 2-fluoroestradiol was prepared by Kurt W. Raack and Kenneth J. Christy. The DMBA-treated rats were kindly provided by Dr. Ellen Rorke.

Appendix A

Calculation of Partition Coefficients: Particular Comments About Steroids

Methods for calculating octanol-water partition coefficients have been described in detail in the literature (Hansch *et al.* 1979; Rekker, 1978). Two basic approaches have been developed, that of Hansch, which is a substitutive method and utilizes substituent constants (π values) which represent the contribution of a particular group or substituent to the partition coefficient of a molecule, and that of Rekker, which is a fragment approach and utilizes molecular fragments (f) that are summed to give the partition coefficient of the whole molecule. In both cases, the π and f values are derived empirically from the measured partition coefficients of a large number of model compounds. With many classes of compounds, the additivity relationships of these substituents or fragments hold nicely, so that partition coefficients for whole molecules can be calculated simply by summation of substituents or fragments.

The additivity relationships of the π and f values, however, appear to work less successfully in predicting the partition coefficients of large, rigid, crowded, lipophilic molecules such as steroids and steroid analogs. Table 4 lists the calculated and measured values for the partition coefficients for whole molecules can be calculated simply discrepancy between measured and calculated values is large. However, in our use of the log P values to estimate the level of nonspecific binding relative to that of estradiol (NSB), it is important only to know the log P of a compound relative to that of estradiol. Therefore, in this report, we have used the values of log P determined experimentally for the parent compounds estradiol, hexestrol, and diethylstilbestrol, and we have caclulated the log P values of their derivatives by addition or subtraction of the appropriate substituent values (π)

TABLE IV
Calculated and Measured Values for the Octanol-Water
Partition Coefficients of Steroids and Non-Steroidal Estrogens

	Log P	
Compound	Calculated[a]	Experimental
17β-Estradiol	4.95	3.97[b]
Hexestrol	5.52	4.24[b]
Diethylstilbestrol	5.22	4.20[b]
Dimethylstilbestrol	4.22	4.05[b]
Testosterone	3.78	3.32[c]
Progesterone	4.67	3.91[b]

[a] Using Hansch's π values (Table V).

[b] Determined in our laboratory

[c] Obtained from Leo *et al.,* (1971)

A basic set of values for the substituents of interest to us is given in Table V. Included in this table are the contributions due to branching, folding, and ring closure, and the effect that each contribution will have on NSB (calculated from equation 5) is given in parentheses.

Where it is appropriate, we have chosen to use more specifically-defined π values for halogen substituents ortho to a phenolic hydroxyl group (Table VI). The folding contribution is encountered when a group (X) is situated as in $PhCH_2CH_2CH_2X$; the log P value is decreased due to interaction of the dipole of the group as it folds back upon the aromatic π system. This is the situation with the side chain halogenated hexestrols, and in these cases, we have used the folding contributions for the individual halogens (Table VII), rather than the average factor given in Table V.

TABLE V

Substituent Contributions (π) to the 1-Octanol:Water
Partition Coefficient (Log P)[a]

Substituent	π aromatic[b] (SA)[c]	π aliphatic[b] (SA)[c]

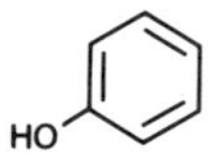		1.46
CH_3-, $-CH_2-$ $CH-$, $-C-$		0.5　(2.4)
Branching in carbon chain		- 0.2　(0.71)
Branching in functional group		- 0.2　(0.71)
Ring Closure		- 0.09　(0.93)
Double Bond		- 0.3　(0.60)
Folding		- 0.6　(0.36)
Intramolecular Hydrogen Bond		0.65　(3.0)
ring joining[d]		- 0.20
- F	0.14　(1.25)	- 0.17　(0.75)
- Cl	0.71　(3.4)	0.39　(1.9)
- Br	0.86　(4.5)	0.60　(2.8)
- I	1.12　(6.9)	1.00　(5.6)
- OH	- 0.67　(0.32)	- 1.16　(0.14)
- OCH_3	- 0.02　(0.96)	- 0.47　(0.45)
- CO_2CH_3	- 0.01　(1.0)	- 0.27　(0.63)

[a] From Leo *et al.*, (1971)

[b] These are average values. For the effect of substituent position in phenolic rings or folding of alkylphenyl groups, see Tables VI and VII.

[c] Effect of substituent on serum albumin binding; calculated from equation 5.

[d] From Rekker (1978).

TABLE VI

π Values for Groups Ortho to a Phenolic Hydroxyl Group[a]

Group	π Value
F	0.25
Cl	0.69
Br	0.89
I	1.19

[a] From Hansch *et al.*, (1973)

TABLE VII

Effect of Folding[a]

X	$\Delta \pi$
OH	- 0.64
F	- 0.56
Cl	- 0.52
Br	- 0.56
I	- 0.78

[a] From Leo *et al.,* (1971).

Substituent values for an aliphatic ethynyl group and an aromatic carbonyl group that were needed to calculate the log P values for the compounds in Table 2 have not been published. The method we have used to estimate these values are outlined below:

6-oxo-estradiol

$$\log P = \log P (E_2) - \pi (CH_3)_{ar} + \pi (C{=}O)_{ar}$$
$$= 3.97 - (0.56) + (- 1.05)*$$
$$= 2.36$$

$\pi (C{=}O)_{ar}$ is derived from $\pi_{ar} (\overset{\overset{O}{\|}}{C}{-}CH_3) - \pi_{ar}(CH_3)$ (Rekker , 1978)

17α-ethynylestradiol

A π value of 0.40 is given for $(\text{-}CH{\equiv}CH)_{ar}$ in Rekker, (1978). To this is added the difference (0.27) between the π_{al} and π_{ar} values of $C{\equiv}N$. Therefore, $\pi_{al} (\text{-}C{\equiv}CH)$ becomes 0.67.

References

Allison, K. J. and Katzenellenbogen, J. A. (1980). In preparation.

Anderson, J. N., Peck, E. J. Jr., and Clark, J. H. (1974). *J. Steroid Biochem.* 5, 103.

Blondeau, J.-P. and Robel P. (1975). *Eur. J. Biochem.* 55, 375.

Blondeau, J.-P., Rocher, P., and Robel, P. (1978). *Steroids.* 32, 563.

Bucourt, R., Vignau, M., Torelli, V., Richard-Foy, H., Geynet, G., Secco-Millet, C., Redeuilh, G., Baulieu, E. E. (1978). *J. Biol. Chem.* 253, 8221.

Carlson, K. E., Sun, L.-H., and Katzenellenbogen, J. A. (1977). *Biochemistry* 16, 4288.

Carlson, R. M., Carlson, R. E., and Kopperman, H. L. (1975). *J. Chromatogr.* 107, 219.

Dandliker, W. B., Brawn, R. J., HSU, N-L., Brawn, P. N., Levin, J., Meyers, C. Y. and Kolb, V. N. (1978). *Cancer Res.* 38, 4212.

36   J.A. Katzenellenbogen et al.

Goswami, R., Heiman, D. F., Harsy, S. G., and Katzenellenbogen, J. A. (1980). *J. Med. Chem.* **23**. In Press.

Hähnel, R. and Twaddle, E. (1979). *J. Steroid Biochem.* **10**, 95.

Hansch, C., Kiehs, K., Lawrence, G. L. (1965). *J. Amer. Chem. Soc.* **87**, 5770.

Hansch, C., Leo, A., Unger, S. H., Kim, K. H., Nikaitani, D., and Lien, E. J. (1973). *J. Med. Chem.* **16**, 1207.

Hansch, C. and Leo, A. (1979). *"Substituent Constants for Correlation Analysis"* Wiley Interscience, New York.

Heiman, D. F., Katzenellenbogen, J. A., and Neeley, R. J. (1980). *J. Med. Chem.* **23**, In Press.

Helmer, F., Kiehs, K., and Hansch, C. (1968). *Biochemistry* **7**, 2858.

Jensen, E. V. and Jacobson, H. I. (1968). *Recent Progr. Horm. Res.* **18**, 387.

Katzenellenbogen, J. A., Johnson, H. J., Jr., and Myers, H. N. (1973). *Biochemistry* **12**, 4085.

Katzenellenbogen, J. A., Johnson, H. J., Jr., and Carlson, K. E. (1973). *Biochemistry* **12**, 4092.

Katzenellenbogen, J. A., Hsuing, H. M., Carlson, K. E., McGuire, W. L., Kraay, R. J., and Katzenellenbogen, B. S. (1975). *Biochemistry* **14**, 1742.

Katzenellenbogen, J. A., Carlson, K. E., Johnson, H. J., Jr., and Myers, H. N. (1977). *Biochemistry* **16**, 1970.

Katzenellenbogen, J. A. (1977). *In* "Biochemical Actions of Hormones" (G. Litwak, ed.), Vol. **4**, p. 1. Academic Press, New York.

Katzenellenbogen, J. A. (1978). *Fed. Proc.* **37**, 174.

Katzenellenbogen, J. A., Carlson, K. E., Heiman, D. F., and Goswami, R. (1980). *J. Nucl Med.* **21** (Submitted for publication).

Komai, T., Eckelman, W. C., Johnsonbaugh, R. E., Mazaitis, A, Kubota, H., and Reba, R. C. (1977). *J. Nucl. Med.* **18**, 360.

Lee, S. H. (1978). *Amer. J. Clin. Path.* **70**, 197.

Lee, Y. J., Notides, A C., Tsay, Y-G., and Kende, A. S. (1977). *Biochemistry* **16**, 2896.

Leo, A., Hansch, C., Elkins, D. (1971). *Chem Rev.* **71**, 525.

Levitzki, A., Sevila, N., Atlas, D., and Steer, M. L. (1975). *J. Mol. Biol.* **97**, 35.

McCall, J. M. (1975). *J. Med. Chem.* **18**, 549.

McGuire, W. L., Horwitz, K. B., Zava, D. T., Garola, R. T., and Chamness, G. C. (1978). *Metabolism* **27**, 287.

Mirrlees, M. S., Moulton, S. J., Murphy, C. T., and Taylor, P. J. (1976). *J. Med. Chem.* **19**, 615.

Payne, D. W. and Katzenellenbogen, J. A., (1979). *Endocrinology* **105**, 743.

Perlman, W. H., Fong, I. F. F., and Tou, J. H. (1969). *J. Biol. Chem.* **244**, 1373.

Pertschuk, L. P., Zava, D. T., Gaetjens, E., Macchia, R. J., Brigati, D. J. and Kim, D. S. (1978). *Res. Commun. Chem. Pathol. Pharmacol.* **22**, 427.

Raynaud, J. P., Bouton, M. M., Gallet-Bourquin, D., Philibert, D., Tournamine, C., and Azadian-Bourlanger, G. (1973). *Molec. Pharmac.* **9**, 520.

Raynaud, J. P., Martin, P. M., Bouton, M. M., and Ojasso, T. (1978). *Cancer Res.* **38**, 3044.

Rekker, R. F. (1978). *"The Hydrophobic Fragmental Constant"* Elsevier North Holland, New York.

Richard-Foy, H., Redeuilh, G., and Richard-Foy, R. (1978). *Anal. Biochem.* **88**, 367.

Scatchard, G. (1949). *Ann. N. Y. Acad. Sci.* **51**, 660.

Sica, V., Parikh, I., Nola, E., Puca, G. A., and Cuatrecasas, P. (1973). *J. Biol. Chem.* **248**, 6543.

Stancel, G. M. and Gorski, J. (1975). *Methods in Enzymology* **36**, 166.
Tsai, T-L.S., and Katzenellenbogen, B. S. (1977). *Cancer Res.* **37**, 1537.
Unger, S. H., Cook, J. R., and Hollenberg, J. S. (1978). *J. Pharm. Sci.* **67**, 136.
Westphal, U. (1971). *"Steroid Protein Interacions"*. Springer Verlag New York.
Zaagsma, J., Meems, L., and Boorsma, M. (1977). *Arch. Pharmacol.* **298**, 29.

Discussion

Wittliff: I am a little bit puzzled by something that we observed with human tumors. There are many human breast tumors that show enormous quantities of non specific binding due to the inclusion of necrotic material in the sample that is assayed. About 70 or 80% of the titration curve can be attributed to non specific binding and yet the dissociation constant of many of these are 10^{-11} molar with only 15 or 20 femtomoles bound per mg of cytosol protein. I am trying to rationalize this with the statement you made about the lamb uterine receptor.

Katzenellenbogen: Are you using estradiol to do the affinity measurements ?

Wittliff: Yes.

Katzenellenbogen: The extent to which non specific binding interferes with the estimates of specific binding is accentuated by the lipophilicity of the compound involved. In fact we became aware of this when we started investigating some very lipophilic compounds, particularly the iodinated ones and the ortho substituted hexestrols. I assume also that in doing your Scatchard measurements you haven't made the correction, that is the $1 + nk$ division, to correct the level of free compound.

Wittliff: Not the way you made the correction.

Katzenellenbogen : The affinities may in fact be higher than your measurement if you include a correction like this. If you have sufficient tissue it is really just a matter of making a three point curve by equilibrium dialysis.
  You can minimize the extent to which non-specific binding will perturb your receptor affinity measurement simply by diluting the cytosol to the maximum extent you can do and still get reasonable estimates of binding.

Zeelen: I fully support your idea of the merit factor. Intuitively you would expect it to be strongly dependent on the temperature. Do you have any experience on that ?

Katzenellenbogen: The temperature is certainly going to be a factor and binding affinities are in this case quite temperature-dependent, although I cannot tell you what these quantitatively are. So that is one aspect we will have to deal with in refining the merit factor concept. Another deficiency of the merit factor, which I may just mention, is that we have defined it in terms of equilibrium binding. If you are looking for an agent which will image a breast tumor, the kinetic factors are going to be very important. Your imaging compound will clear faster from the rapidly dissociating sites and less rapidly from the receptor sites. Therefore kinetic factors will be the important ones in terms of the biological or the *in vivo* distribution.

STRUCTURE-ACTIVITY RELATIONSHIPS
OF STEROID ESTROGENS

F. J. ZEELEN AND E. W. BERGINK

Organon, Scientific Development Group
5340 BH Oss, The Netherlands

Introduction

Research in recent years has shown that estrogens bind to specific proteins (receptors) in target organs (Jensen *et al.*, 1966). Formation of an estrogen-protein complex in the cytoplasm of sensitive cells is the first and essential step for the hormonal effects to be realised. We discuss in this paper the relationship between the chemical structure and binding to the rabbit uterine estrogen receptor. Binding affinities were determined using a competition assay with [^{3}H] - estradiol and dextran-coated charcoal adsorption [Appendix].

Using Free-Wilson analysis, Fanchenko *et al.* (1979) showed that the contribution of substituents to binding is independent of the presence of other groups indicating that all steroid estrogens bind at approx. the same position. This makes it possible to estimate the contribution to binding of the individual substituents.

Which factors are important for binding ?

The two functional groups of the estradiol molecule, the 3-OH and 17-OH group, play an important role in binding. It has even been suggested that the rest of the molecule only serves as a spacer to hold these two groups at the right distance (Schueler, 1946; Grundy, 1957). It can be calculated, however, from the binding data in Fig. 1 that at 4°C each of the hydroxyl functions contributes about 8 kJ/mole (2 kcal/mole), leaving for the contribution of the steroid skeleton about 34 kJ/mole (8 kcal/mole). These values for the hydroxyl groups are in the right order of magnitude for hydrogen bonds. We

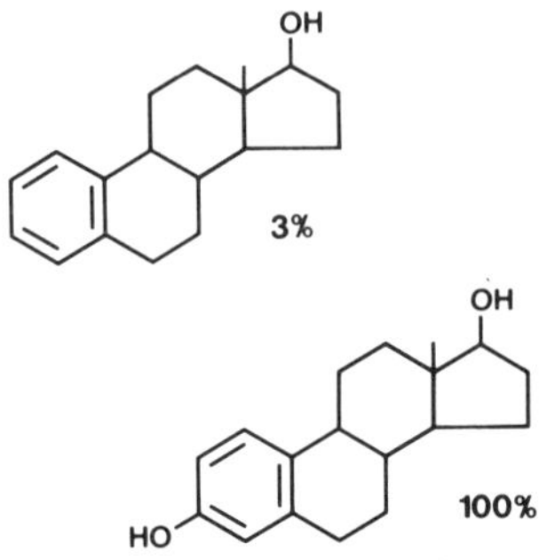

Fig. 1: Importance of the functional groups for the binding of estradiol.

conclude from these data that the steroid skeleton contributes more to binding than the two functional groups. This is also illustrated by the enantiomer of estradiol, which has exactly the same distance between the two hydroxyl groups. For the rabbit uterine receptor we found that the enantiomer had only 4% the affinity of estradiol which is in close agreement with reported data (Chernayaev et al., 1975). Two effects may be important for the binding of the steroid skeleton to the receptor: hydrophobic binding and π -complex formation with the aromatic ring. Attempts to separate these two effects by direct measurement of the entropy change during binding has given contradicting results (Lövgren et al., 1978; Sanborn et al., 1971). We have shown the importance of π -complex formation with the aromatic ring (Fig. 2). Although the hydrophobicity of the two compounds is of the same order of magnitude, the aromatic compound shows a much stronger binding.

In line with this is our finding that the binding of thiophene analogues is similar to that of the corresponding benzene parent compound (Fig. 3)*.

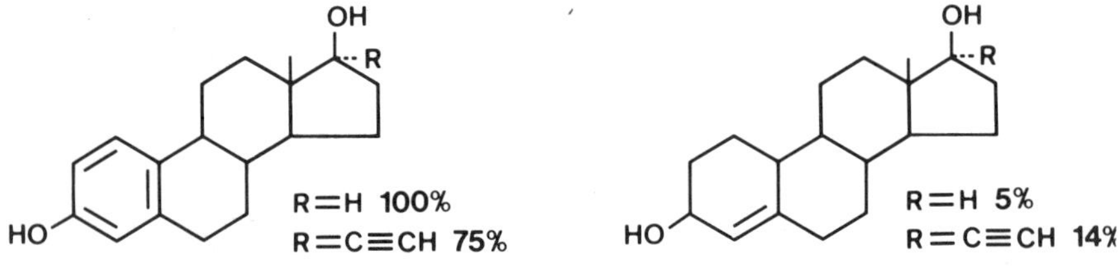

Fig. 2: Importance of the aromatic ring for binding

* We thank Prof. Buck and Dr. Corvers, Technical University Eindhoven, for making available these compounds for testing.

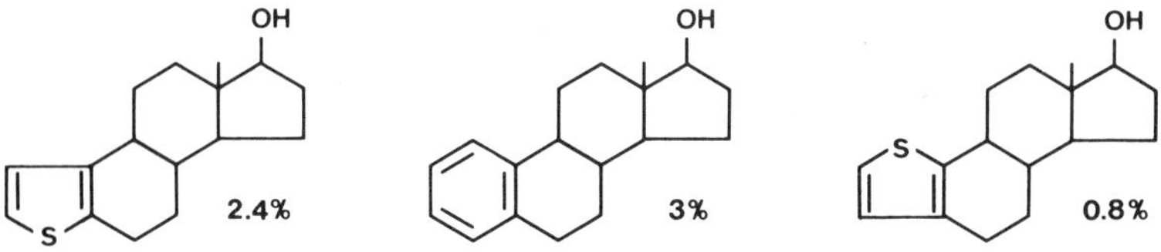

Fig. 3: Binding of thiophene analogues*

It follows however from the data given that the contribution of the aromatic ring to the total binding energy is only some 4 kJ/mole (1 kcal/mole) so that hydrophobic binding between the steroid skeleton and the protein must be the most important factor. This is illustrated by the following example. Fachenko *et al.* (1979) reported that replacement of the ring 11-methylene group by a polar 11-aza group leads to greatly reduced binding. It also explains why 8-azaestradiol and 8-azaestrone displayed very low estrogenic activity despite the fact that the X-ray structure analysis showed these compounds to have exactly the same dimensions as estradiol and estrone respectively (Brown *et al.*, 1971; Majeste *et al.*, 1969). We found that the introduction of double bonds, which generally leads to a decrease in hydrophobicity (a decreased tendency to leave the aqueous phase), tends to decrease affinity for the receptor (Table I).

TABLE I

Relative binding of unsaturated estradiol analogues

Position additional double bonds	Relative affinity
none	100 %
6- 7	28 %
9-11	12 %
7- 8	82 %
6- 7 and 8- 9	18 %

Estrogens as carriers of cytotoxic groups

It follows from the above discussion that if one plans to use the steroid molecule as a cytotoxic group carrier to fight estrogen-dependant tumors that the cytotoxic groups should be as hydrophobic as possible and should not be attached to the 3 or 17 positions

* The thiophines were racemates. The figures given are based on the assumption that only the natural isomer contributes to binding.

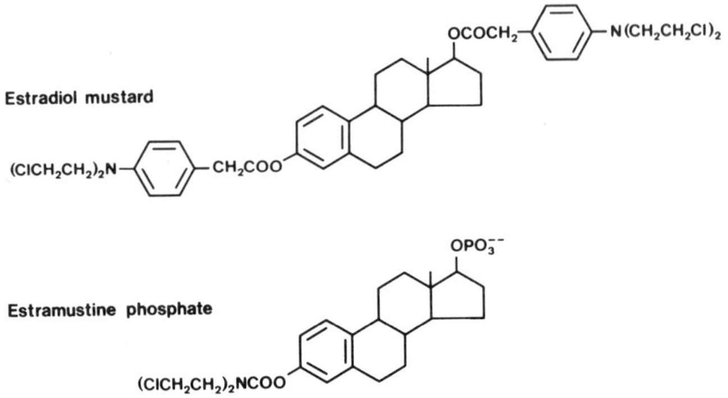

Fig. 4: Estradiol derivatives with very low affinity for the estrogen receptor

as this will lead to greatly reduced binding. This is confirmed by the study of Wittliff *et al.*, (1978) showing that estradiol mustard and estramustine phosphate (Fig. 4) have a very low affinity (1/10 000 that of estradiol) for the estrogen receptor.

For the same reason we expect that the nitrosourea derivatives recently reported by Lam *et al.*, (1979) will also show low affinity for the estrogen receptor.

In order to find more suitable positions in the estradiol molecule for substitution with cytotoxic groups, we used a methyl group as a probe. This group is so hydrophobic that under ideal conditions (no steric interference with binding) it will increase binding energy by about 4 kJ/mole (1 kcal/mole) and produce binding, which is 600 % that of estradiol. We may thus expect to find affinities that can be determined easily.

Although the effect of the hydrophobic methyl group would have been more pronounced at 37°C measurements were done at 4°C in view of the limited stability of the receptor at higher temperatures. Some of the chosen derivatives were synthesized using partial synthesis, while for others a biomimetic total synthesis was used (Groen *et al.*, 1978). We found that positions where the introduction of a methyl group leads to low or moderate affinity are the 1 (15 %), 2 (36 %), 6α (31 %), 15α (rac. 29 %), 15β (26 %) and 18 (31 %) position. Raynaud (1979) has reported similar results for the mouse uterine receptor for the 2 (41 %), 9α (39 %) and 18 (31 %) methyl derivatives.

Positions where the introduction of a methyl group leads to a relatively high affinity are the 7α (104 %), 11β (65 %) and 17α (83 %) positions. For the mouse (Raynaud, 1979) high affinity was reported

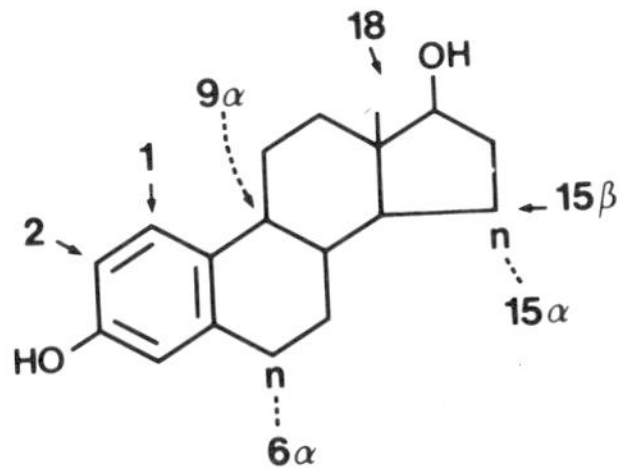

Fig. 5: Positions in the estradiol molecule, where methyl substitution leads to greatly reduced affinity for the rabbit uterine estrogen receptor.

for the 7α (101 %) and 12β (111 %) methyl derivatives. In no case however was the affinity significantly higher than that of estradiol suggesting that the effect of increased hydrophobic binding was counteracted by the effect of steric hindrance. To study this further we varied the substituents at the 7α-position (Table II).

TABLE II
Relative affinity of 7α-substituted estradiols

substituent	relative affinity
H	100 %
CH_3	104 %
OH	0,9 %
CH_2OCH_3	28 %

These data show that substitution of a hydrophobic group like a methyl group is tolerated but that hydrophilic groups like the hydroxyl group greatly reduce binding affinity. This indicates that the active site of the receptor is strongly lipophilic. Relative to estradiol, 7α-methylestradiol had a 104 % binding at 4°C but had a 160 % binding at 30°C. This confirms that hydrophobic interactions are important here. Results for the 11β-position are comparable (Table III) with those for the 7α-position. Low affinity was also found for the 15α-hydroxy derivatives of estradiol. Based on a quantitative study on the relationship between structure and binding affinity for the rat uterine receptor of a series of 16α-substituted estradiol derivatives. Ponsold, Draffehn and Schönecker (1977) concluded that also for this position hydrophobic interactions led to an increased and steric hindrance to a decreased affinity.

In the present study we selected the 11β-position for the introduction of a cytotoxic group and synthesized two aziridine derivatives (Fig. 6). The binding of these compounds is low compared to estra-

TABLE III
Relative affinity of 11β-substituted estradiols

substituent	relative affinity
H	100 %
C_2H_5	78 %
CH_3	65 %
CH_2OCH_3	37 %
OH	7 %

diol but high in comparison to other known cytotoxic steroids. These compounds are now being evaluated for anti-cancer activity.

Discussion

The presented data suggest that in the estrogen-receptor complex the steroid is tightly surrounded by the protein. In order to accomodate substituents the protein has to be distorted. The energy needed for this process leads to reduced affinity, unless it can be compensated for by increased hydrophobic binding. Our results give no indication of the existence of special hydrophobic pockets on the receptor for 7α-or 18-substituents on the estradiol molecule as suggested by Durani et al., (1979). Some parts of the protein appear to be more flexible than others, so that some positions of the estradiol molecule tolerate substitution better than others. The non-planar diethylstilbestrol or even the 14β, 17α-isomer of estradiol (Fig. 7) still show reasonable affinity. In contrast to the progesterone receptor where both hydrophobic and hydrophilic areas can be distinguished (Lee et al., 1977), the active site of the estradiol receptor seems to be only hydrophobic.

Using affinity chromatography Bucourt et al., (1978) showed that at the 7α- or 17α-position, a spacer consisting of a chain of at least 14 atoms was necessary to penetrate the protein surrounding the

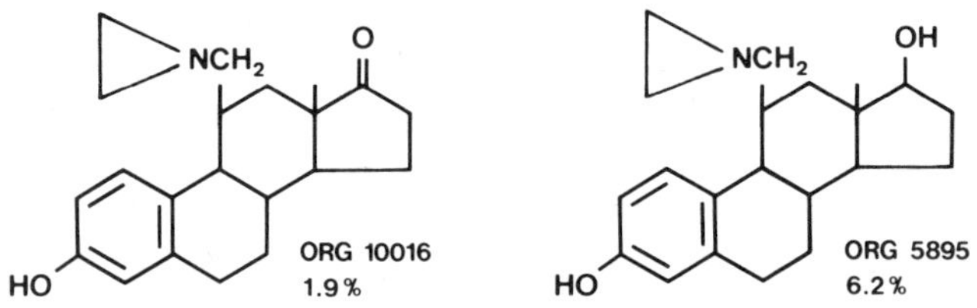

Fig. 6: Relative affinities of aziridine derivatives of estradiol.

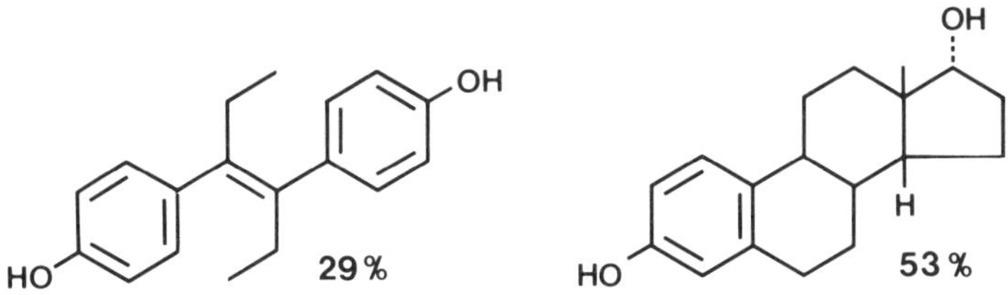

Fig. 7: Affinity of two non planar derivatives.

estradiol molecule. We estimated the thickness of the surrounding protein to be $15\text{-}20 \times 10^{-10}$ m, large in comparison with for example the 12×10^{-10} m $O_3\text{-}O_{17}$ distance in the estradiol molecule. It is evident from the proposed model that the complex formation can not be a simple diffussion of the estrogen into a preformed cavity, but that the association should be accompanied by a conformational change in the protein molecule. In agreement with this, the association rate is much lower than that (10^9 litres moles $^{-1}\text{sec}^{-1}$) expected for a diffusion-controlled process (Burgen, 1966; Stroupe *et al.*, 1975) and the energy of activation of about 50 kJ/mole (12 kcal/mole) is much higher than the 17 kJ/mole (4 kcal/mole) expected for a diffusion-controlled process.

Acknowledgement

We thank M. S. de Winter for constructive criticism and stimulating discussions.

References

Brown, J. N., and Trefonas, L. M. (1972). *J. Am. Chem. Soc.*, **94**, 4311.
Bucourt, R., Vignau, M., Torelli, V., Richard-Foy, H., Geynet, C., Secco-Millet, C., Redeuilh, G. and Baulieu, E. E. (1978). *J. Biol. Chem.* **253**, 8221.
Burgen, A. S. V. (1966). *J. Pharm. Pharmacol.*, **18**, 137.
Chernayaev, G. A., Barkova, T. I., Egorova, V. V., Sorokina, I. B., Ananchenko, S. N., Mataradze, G. D., Sokolova, I. B. and Rozen, V. B. (1975), *J. Steroid. Biochem.* **6**, 1483.
Durani, S., Agarwal, A. K., Saxena, R., Setty, B. S., Gupta, R. C., Kole, P. L., Ray, S. and Anand, N. (1979). *J. Steroid. Biochem.*, **11**, 67.
Fanchenko, N. D., Sturchak, S. V., Schchedrina, R. N., Pivnitsky, K. K., Novikov, E. A. and Ishkov, V. L. (1979). *Acta endocr.* (Kbh) **90**, 167.
Groen, M. B., van Vliet, N. P. and Zeelen, F. J. (1978). *In Plenary Lectures 11th International Symposium on Chemistry of Natural Products*, Vol. IV, 2, p. 380. Bulgarian Academy of Sciences, Sofia.
Grundy, J. (1957). *Chem. Rev.*, **57**, 305.
Jensen, E. V., Jacobsen, H. J., Flescher, J. W., Saha, N. N., Gupta, G. N., Smith,

S., Colucci, V., Shiplacoff, D., Neumann, H. G., DeSombre, E. R. and Jong-blut, P. W. (1966). *In Steroid Dynamics*, p. 133. Academic Press, New York.

Lam, H. Y. P., Begleiter, A., Goldenberg, G. J. and Wong, C. M. (1979). *J. Med. Chem.*, **22**, 200.

Lee, D. L., Kollmann, P. A., Marsh, F. J. and Wolff, M. E. (1977). *J. Med. Chem.*, **20**, 1139.

Lörgen, T., Pettersson, K., Kouvonen, I. and Punnonen, R. (1978). *J. Steroid. Biochem.*, **9**, 803.

Majeste, R. and Trefonas, L. M. (1969). *J. Am. Chem. Soc.*, **91**, 1508.

Ponsold, K., Draffehn, J. and Schönecker, B. (1977). *Pharmazie* **32**, 596.

Raynaud, J. P. (1979). *In Drug Design VIII* (E. J. Ariens ed.), p. 182, Academic Press, New York.

Sanborn, B. M., Ramanath Rao, B. and Korenman, S. G. (1971). *Biochemistry* **10**, 4955.

Schueler, F. W. (1946). *Science*, **103**, 221.

Stroupe, S. D. and Westphal, U. (1975). *J. Biol. Chem.*, **250**, 8735.

Witliff, J. L., Weidner, N., Everson, R. B. and Hall, T. C. (1978). *Cancer Treatment Reports* **62**, 1262.

Material and Methods

Material

$[6.7-^3H]$-estradiol-17β (90 Ci/mmole) was manufactured by the Radiochemical Centre, Amersham, Great Britain. Microtitration plates (system Cooke, type M 220-29AR), were obtained from Greiner, West Germany. The tissue homogenizer, Polytron type PT 10-35, was made by Kinematica, Switzerland. The centrifuge, which was used for the dextrancoated charcoal procedure, was a Sorvall type RC-3 with special holders for the microtitration plates.

Animals

Female Dutch (belted) rabbits, aged 6 months, were obtained from the Broekman Institute, Stiphout, The Netherlands. They were ovariectomized and kept for a predosing period of 1 week before being treated daily for 7 days with a subcutaneous dose of 10 μg estradiol-17β (100 μg/ml arachis oil). The animals were killed 24 hours after the last injection with an overdose of nembutal and exsanguinated via the carotid arteries. The uterus was excised immediately, the endometrium was removed and the myometrium was stored in liquid nitrogen.

Competitive binding studies

All procedures were carried out at 4°C. The frozen myometrium was cut up and homogenized in 5 volumes (v/w) of TE buffer (10 mM Tris-HCl, 1 mM EDTA, 0.5 mM dithioerythritol 0.002 % NaN_3, pH

7,4). The cytosol fraction was obtained after centrifugation of the homogenate for 20 minutes at 110 000 g and aliquots (0.100 ml) were added to the wells of the microtitration plates and incubated with 7 nM [^{3}H]-estradiol-17β and increasing concentrations (low, medium and high; ratio of molarities 1:2:4) of the unlabeled test steroids for either 18 h at 4°C or 18 h at 4°C and subsequently 1.5 h at 30°C. The selection of the concentration range for the competitor was such that, if possible, 50% of the initially bound [^{3}H]-estradiol-17β remained bound in the presence of the medium concentration of the competitor. Non specific binding sites were assessed with 50-fold excess of the unlabeled estradiol-17β. Unbound ligand was removed by incubating (with continuous shaking for 5 min) the mixture with 0.100 ml dextran-coated charcoal suspension (0.25 % charcoal, 0.025 % dextran T70 in TE buffer). The microtitration plates were centrifuged at 1500 g for 5 min and 0.100 ml of the supernatant was added to 9 ml scintillation fluid and counted in the Packard Liquid Scintillation counter. The parallel line assay of Rodbard and Lewald using ln B/(B$_t$-B), was chosen to calculate the relative affinities of the unlabeled steroids.

Reference

Rondbard, D, and Lewald, J. E., (1970). *Acta Endocrinol. Suppl.* **147**, 79-99.

Discussion

Blickenstaff: You said that an 11-β methyl group gives a binding of 65% and an 11-β ethyl group 78% (estradiol 100%). This makes me wonder if there is a particular hydrophobic pocket at 11-β. Do you see any merit in exploring that pocket by putting on larger alkyl groups?

Zeelen: I don't believe that our data support the idea of a specific pocket. If there is a specific pocket so that the methyl group can stick in and undergo hydrophobic interaction without disturbing the protein molecule, you would expect an increase in binding energy of roughly 1 kcal/mole, which means a binding affinity of 600%. However only 65% is observed, meaning that the gain in binding energy from hydrophobic interaction has to be neutralized by the energy required for the distortion of the molecule. Putting in an ethyl group increases the hydrophobic interaction by another 1 kcal/mole and requires a smaller extra distortion of the protein molecule (binding affinity 78%).

So I don't see any reason to assume a particular hydrophobic pocket.

Konives: Do you have any experience with compounds having a nitrogen not directly attached to the steroid ring, for example through a connecting group?

Zeelen: The only one we synthesized was the one with the aziridine ring in 11-β, where the nitrogen was connected to the steroid through a methylene group. Here indeed we see reasonable but still very low binding. I have no other examples.

Hamacher: The introduction of polar groups in the hydrophobic site of the steroid decreases the affinity for the receptor. In the last part of your presentation you discussed the possibility of introducing spacers between polar groups and these sites.

How long do you think a spacer chain should be to preserve the affinity for the receptor ?

Zeelen: We think that if you want to have your steroid attached polar group sticking through the protein surrounding in the water, you need at least 14-15 carbon atoms in your connecting chain. This was clearly demonstrated by Bucourt *et al.* in their paper on affinity chromatography of the receptor.

THE DESIGN OF ESTROGENS AND/OR ANTI-ESTROGENS ON THE BASIS OF RECEPTOR BINDING

J. P. RAYNAUD* AND M. M. BOUTON

Centre de Recherches Roussel-Uclaf, 93230 Romainville, France

Introduction

The need for new, more powerful, and better tolerated anti-estrogens has become increasingly evident since it has been shown that they can be used to treat hormone-dependent cancers with some success. The present paper describes a simple method for the selection of such compounds on the basis of their relative binding affinities for cytosolic steroid hormone receptors.

Compounds like tamoxifen, nafoxidine, CI 628, estriol, dimethyl-stilbestrol or RU 16117, which antagonize the development of artificially-induced mammary tumors (Desombre *et al.*, 1974; Jordan, 1976; Kelly *et al.*, 1977; Nicholson *et al.*, 1975; Terenius, 1971), also antagonize estradiol-induced responses. It has been suggested that their anti-estrogenic activity results from an interaction with the cytosolic estrogen receptor with which they form rapidly dissociating complexes (Bouton *et al.*, 1979; Capony *et al.*, 1977 & 1978; Katzenellenbogen *et al.*, 1978). To confirm this hypothesis, we have attempted to relate the anti-estrogenic potency of a series of compounds with the kinetics of their binding to the estrogen receptor, as measured by their relative binding affinities under different incubation conditions (Bouton *et al.*, 1978).

---

*This paper was not fully discussed during the workshop because J. P. Raynaud was unable to attend. The crystallographic part of the work and the receptor binding data were presented by M. Hospital.

Testosterone, progesterone and certain progestins (e.g. medroxy-progesterone acetate, norgestrel; norethisterone) also inhibit the estradiol-induced increase in uterine weight (Lerner, 1974; Raynaud *et al.*, 1979). It has been suggested that the anti-estrogenic activity of progesterone, which does not bind to the estrogen receptor (Black *et al.*, 1973; Di Carlo *et al.*, 1978; Raynaud *et al.*, 1979; Watson *et al.*, 1977), could be due to inhibition of cytosolic estrogen receptor replenishment (Bhakoo *et al.*, 1977; Clark *et al.*, 1977). Since this inhibition is characteristic of progesterone (testosterone has only a slight inhibitory effect, whereas cortisol has none (Bhakoo *et al.*, 1977; Clark *et al.*, 1977), we have compared the ability of several progestins to inhibit estrogen receptor replenishment in order to establish whether this property is related to anti-estrogenic activity and to binding to the cytosolic progestin receptor and whether binding to the progestin receptor could be considered a criterion for anti-estrogenic activity.

Material and methods

Animals

Immature (18 day-old) or castrated adult (7 weeks) female mice (Swiss Strain) and adult male rats (Sprague Dawley) were purchased from Iffa-Credo (France). Immature female rabbits (New-Zealand) were purchased from Charles River (France).

Test compounds

[6,7 ^{3}H] Estradiol (53.6 Ci/mmole), [6,7 ^{3}H] moxestrol (52 Ci/mmole), [6,7 ^{3}H] RU 16117 (46 Ci/mmole), [6,7 ^{3}H] promegestone (55.4 Ci/mmole) and [6,7 ^{3}H] metribolone (55.5 Ci/mmole) were synthesized at the Roussel-Uclaf Research Centre and checked for purity ($\geqslant 95\%$) by thin-layer chromatography before use. Unlabeled steroids (see Table I) were synthesized at the Roussel-Uclaf Research Centre, compound J 60 (RU 26143) in the laboratory of Professor J. Jacques (Collège de France, Paris) and compound C 7701 in the laboratory of Dr. J. F. Miquel (Laboratoires du C.N.R.S., C.E.R.C.O.A., Thiais, France).

Cytosol preparation

Uteri from immature mice or from estrogen-primed rabbits were homogenized in 1/50 (w/v) of TS buffer (10 mM Tris-HCl, pH 7.4, 0.25 M sucrose) with a moter-driven all-glass conic homogenizer. Prostates from castrated rats were homogenized in 1/5 (w/v) of TS

TABLE I
Chemical names of test-substances

1. Compounds that bind to the estrogen receptor :

Estradiol	Estra-1,3,5(10)-triene-3,17β-diol
Estriol	Estra-1,3,5(10)-trienne-3,16α,17β-triol
Ethynyl estradiol	19-Nor-17α-pregna-1,3,5(10)-trien-20-yne-3,17β-diol
2-Methyl estradiol	2-Methyl-estra-1,3,5(10)-triene-3,17β-diol
Moxestrol (RU 2858)	11β-Methoxy-19-nor-17α-pregna-1,3,5(10)-trien-20-yne-3,17β-diol
Nafoxidine (U 11100)	1-[2-[4-(3,4 dihydro-6-methoxy-2-phenyl-1-naphthalenyl)phenyoxy]ethyl)pyrrolidine hydrochloride
RU 15864	3-Hydroxy-17α-hydroxymethyl-estra-1,3,5(10)-triene
RU 16117	11α-Methoxy-19-nor-17α-pregna-1,3,5(10)-trien-20-yne-3,17β-diol
RU 2504	11β-Methoxy-estra-1,3,5(10)-triene-3,17β-diol
RU 26143 (J 60)	2α-Ethynyl-5α-A-nor-estrane-2β,17β-diol
RU 27004	2,3,3-Tris-(4-hydroxyphenyl)prop-2-enonitrile
RU 5444	12β-Methyl-19-nor-17α-pregna-1,3,5(10)-trien-20-yne-3,17β-diol
Tamoxifen (ICI 46474)	(z)2-[4-(1,2-Diphenyl-1-butenyl)-phenoxy]-N,N-dimethyl ethanamine

2. Compounds that do not bind to the estrogen receptor :

RU 25051	(17R) 2'-oxydo-spiro[estra-4,9,11-triene-17,5' (1,2)oxathiolan]3-one
RU 3510	17α-Methyl-19-nor-pregn-4-ene-3,20-dione
Norgestrel	13β-Ethyl-17β-hydroxy-18,19-dinor-17α-pregn-4-en-20-yn-3-one
RU 27987	17α-Methyl-17β-((25)2-hydroxy-1-oxo-propyl)estra-4,9-dien-3-one
Promegestone (RU 5020)	17α,21-Dimethyl-19-nor-pregna-4,9-diene-3,20-dione
RU 22779	(17R)2'-Oxydo-spiro[estr-4-ene-17,5'(1,2)-oxathiolan]3-one (γ-lactone)
Demegestone (RU 2453)	17α-Methyl-19-nor-pregna-4,9-diene-3,20-dione
RU 2420	7α,17α-Dimethyl-17β-hydroxy-estra-4,9,11-trien-3-one
Chlormadinone acetate	17α-Acetyloxy-6-chloro-pregna-4,6-diene-3,20-dione
Medroxyprogesterone acetate	17α-Acetyloxy-6α-methyl-pregn-4-ene-3,20-dione
RU 2999	17β-Hydroxy-17α-methyl-2-oxaestra-4,9,11-trien-3-one
Norethindrone	17β-Hydroxy-19-nor-17α-pregn-4-en-20-yn-3-one
Metribolone (RU 1881)	17β-Hydroxy-17α-methyl-estra-4,9,11-trien-3-one

RU 22761	(17R) 2'-Oxydo-spiro[estra-4,6-diene-17,5'(1,2)-oxathiolan]3-one
RU 15182	17α-Ethyl-19-nor-pregna-4,9-diene-3,20-dione
Megestrol acetate	17α-Acetyloxy-6-methyl-pregna-4,6-diene-3,20-dione
RU 4843	17β-Hydroxy-11β-methoxy-19-nor-17α-pregn-4-en-20-yn-3-one
Progesterone	Pregn-4-ene-3,20-dione
RU 1364	17β-Hydroxy-13β-propyl-18,19-dinor-17α-pregn-4-en-20-yn-3-one
RU 25845	16α-Methyl-19-nor-pregn-4-ene-3,20-dione
Gestrinone (RU 2323)	13β-Ethyl-17β-hydroxy-18,19-dinor-pregna-4,9,11-trien-20-yn-3-one
Norgestrienone (RU 2010)	17β-Hydroxy-19-nor-17α-pregna-4,9,11-trien-20-yn-3-one
RU 18964	19-Nor-10α-pregna-4,6-diene-3,20-dione
Trenbolone (RU 2341)	17β-Hydroxy-estra-4,9,11-trien-3-one
RU 2284	4-Chloro-17β-hydroxy-17α-methyl-estra-4,9,11-trien-3-one
RU 27988	17α-Methyl-17β-[(2R)2-hydroxy-1-oxopropyl]estra-4,9-dien-3-one
Triamcinolone acetonide	9α-Fluoro-11β,21-dihydroxy-16α,17α-[1-methyl-ethylidene bis (oxy)]-pregna-1,4-diene-3,20-dione
RU 1285	17β-Hydroxy-13β-propyl-gon-4-en-3-one
Methylandrostanolone	17β-Hydroxy-17α-methyl-5α-androstan-3-one
Methyltestosterone	17β-Hydroxy-17α-methyl-androst-4-en-3-one
Testosterone	17β-Hydroxy-androst-4-en-3-one
5α-Dihydrotestosterone	17β-Hydroxy-5-α-androstan-3-one
RU 1178	11β,21-Dihydroxy-16α-methyl-pregna-1,4-diene-3,20-dione

buffer in a Teflon-glass homogenizer. Cytosol was prepared by centrifuging the homogenates at 105,000 g for 60 min in a Beckmann ultracentrifuge (Spinco L_2 65$_B$-rotor Ti 50).

Dextran-coated charcoal (DCC) adsorption assay

Cytosol was incubated as described in the table and figure legends. After incubation, a 100 μl sample was stirred for 10 min at 0-4°C in a microtiter plate (Greiner plates, System Cooke M220-24 Å) with 100 μl of a DCC suspension (0.625% Dextran 80,000/1.25% Charcoal Norit A) and then centrifuged for 10 min at 800 g at 0-4°C. The concentration of bound radioligand was determined by measuring the radioactivity in an aliquot of supernatant.

Measurement of the relative binding affinity to receptors

Aliquots of 125 μl of cytosol were incubated with 5 nM [^{3}H] estradiol, [^{3}H] promegestone or [^{3}H] metribolone and various concentrations of unlabeled competitor, as described in the table and figure legends. After incubation, bound labeled steroid (B) was measured by the DCC adsorption technique. The ratio B/B_0, where B_0 represents the concentration of bound radioligand in the absence of unlabeled steroid, was plotted against the concentration, of the added unlabeled steroid. The concentration of unlabeled steroid required for a 50% displacement of radioligand from its specific binding sites (after subtraction of non-specific binding) was determined. The ratio of the 50% displacement concentrations for radioligand and competitor gives the relative binding affinity (RBA) of the competitor (Korenman, 1970).

Measurement of rate constants

a) *Association rate of the cytosolic estrogen receptor complex at 0°C* : A 1 nM concentration of labeled estradiol, moxestrol or RU 16117 was added to cytosol maintained at 0°C. Every 5 min for 1 hr after addition of the labeled steroid, a 100 μl aliquot was transferred into 5000 nM unlabeled steroid in a microtiter plate to stop the reaction. Bound radioactivity was determined by the DCC adsorption techique. Association rate (k $_{+1}$) is given by the slope of the line k $_{+1} = (2.3/E_0-R_0)\log ER_0/RE_0$.

b) *Dissociation rate of the cytosolic estrogen receptor complex at 25°C* : Dissociation rate was measured by the isotopic dilution technique. Unlabeled steroid (2500 nM) was added to cytosol previously incubated with 5 nM labeled estradiol, moxestrol or RU 16117 for 15 hr at 0°C. After different times of incubation at 25°C, 100 μl samples were treated with DCC at 0°C in order to determine bound radioactivity. Dissociation rate (k $_{-1}$) is given by the slope of the line k $_{-1} = 2.3 \log B/B_0$ where B_0 and B represent bound steroid at time t = o and time t respectively.

c) *Dissociation rate of the nuclear estrogen receptor complex at 25°C* : Immature female mice were injected s.c. with 25 μCi/ mouse of tritiated estradiol or moxestrol ($\sim$ 0.1 μg/mouse) or with 10 μg/mouse of unlabeled RU 16117 in 0.1 ml of a 10% solution of ethanol in saline and sacrificed 6 hr after the injection. The uteri were immediately frozen in liquid nitrogen, pulverized with a Thermovac, and homogenized with a motor-driven Teflon-glass homogenizer in 5 volumes (w/v) of TKM buffer (50 mM Tris-HCl, pH 7.4, 25 mM KCL, 5 mM Mg2+) containing 2.2 M sucrose. The homogenate was filtered on 6 layers of nylong gauze and washed with 10 volumes of TKM buffer containing 1.7 M sucrose. Nuclei were prepared by ultracentrifugation on 2 M sucrose according to Chauveau *et al.* (1956). They were washed twice with 2 ml of TKM buffer containing 1 M sucrose and resuspended with a Teflon-glass homogenizer in TKM buffer containing 0.25 M sucrose. Minimal cytoplasmic contamination and no deformation of nuclear shape were detected by light microscopy.

Samples of 250 μl of nuclear suspension labeled after injection of radiolabeled estradiol or moxestrol were incubated with 2500 nM of unlabeled steroid under weak agitation. At different time intervals, nuclei were spun down at 800 g x 10 min, washed with 3 x 1 ml TS buffer and dissolved in 0.5 ml Soluene (Packard); their radioactivity was counted.

When unlabeled RU 16117 was injected, the nuclear suspension obtained was incubated with 25 nM of labeled RU 16117 and B_0 (total binding sites) was measured by an exchange assay (2 hr incubation at 30°C) using [^{3}H] moxestrol as radioligand (Bouton *et al.*, 1979).

Measurement of the inhibition of estrogen receptor replenishment

Castrated mice, primed 2 days previously with 1 μg of moxestrol, were injected s.c. with 1 μg of estradiol in 0.1 ml saline containing 10% ethanol, alone or with various doses of test-steroid injected in 0.1 ml of sesame oil containing 5% benzyl alcohol. Animals were sacrificed 24 hr later. Their uteri were cleaned of fat and mesentery, weighed and homogenized in 50 volumes (w/v) of TS buffer. The homogenate was centrifuged at 2000 rpm for 15 min at 0-4°C. In order to eliminate endogenous steroid, supernatant was vortexed with 1/10 (v/v) of a DCC suspension (3.125% Dextran 80,000 - 6.125% Charcoal Norit A) and then centrifuged at 2000 rpm for 15 min. The concentration of estrogen-specific binding sites in the supernatant was measured by an exchange assay using [^{3}H] moxestrol as radioligand (Raynaud *et al.*, 1978). The percentage inhibition of estrogen receptor replenishment was plotted against the dose of steroid injected and the dose required for 50% inhibition was determined.

Measurement of uterotrophic and anti-uterotrophic activities

Immature female mice were injected s.c. with various doses of test-steroid alone (uterotrophic activity) or in combination with a total dose of 0.3 μg estradiol (anti-uterotrophic activity), daily for 3 consecutive days. Controls received solvent only (0.1 ml saline containing 10% ethanol). Animals were sacrificed 24 hr after the last injection; their uteri were removed, cleaned of fat and mesentery and weighed.

Results

I. Compounds that interact with the estrogen receptor.

A. Estrogen receptor interaction kinetics.

Moxestrol and RU 16117 associated at the same rate with the cytosolic estrogen receptor but about 5 to 10 times slower than estradiol (Fig. 1). However, while moxestrol formed a complex which at 25°C dissociated 6 times slower than the estradiol-receptor complex, RU 16117 formed a complex which dissociated 3 times faster than this complex i.e. about 20 times faster than the moxestrol-receptor complex (Fig. 2a and Table 2).

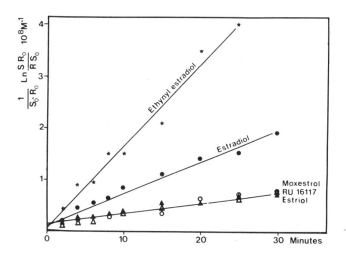

Fig. 1: Association rates of the cytosolic estrogen receptor complexes (0°C) in mouse uterus.

At 25°C, the nuclear complexes obtained 6 hr after injection of steroid dissociated slower than the corresponding cytosolic complexes, but the same ranking was maintained as in the cytosol. The moxestrol nuclear complex dissociated about 20 times slower than the estradiol complex, whereas the RU 16117 nuclear complex dissociated more than 10 times faster than this complex, i.e. about 200 times faster than the moxestrol complex (Fig. 2b and Table 2).

It is possible to compare the kinetics of the interaction of a test-compound with the cytosolic estrogen receptor with estradiol inter-

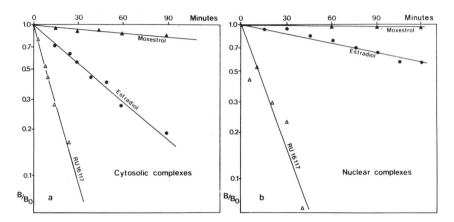

Fig. 2: Dissociation rates of the cytosolic (a) and nuclear (b) steroid receptor complexes (25°C) in mouse uterus.

TABLE II
Dissociation rates of the cytosolic and nuclear steroid-receptor complexes at 25°C

	k_{-1} cytosolic	k_{-1} nuclear
Estradiol	30	8.3
Moxestrol	5	0.4
RU 16117	105	93

k_{-1} is expressed in $\times 10^5 \, \text{sec}^{-1}$

action kinetics by comparing RBA values measured under two sets of appropriately-chosen incubation conditions (e.g. 2 hr at 0°C and 5 hr at 25°C) (Bouton *et al.*, 1978). Thus the compounds in Table I can be classified into 2 categories depending upon whether, like moxestrol, their RBA values increase with incubation time and temperature (e.g. ethynyl estradiol, RU 2504, RU 5444 and C 7701) or, like RU 16117 and estriol, decrease with increasing incubation time and temperature (Table III). By analogy with moxestrol and RU 16117, the former presumably form complexes with the estrogen receptor which dissociate slower than the estradiol-receptor complex, whereas the latter form faster dissociating complexes.

B. Uterotrophic and anti-uterotrophic activities

As shown in Fig. 3, compounds with RBA values increasing with

TABLE III
Relative binding affinities (RBA's) for the cytosolic
estrogen receptor in mouse uterus

	2 hr 0°C		5 hr 25°C	
Ethynyl estradiol	112 ± 5	(9)	245 ± 13	(5)
RU 5444	111 ± 14	(3)	615 ± 99	(3)
C 7701	41 ± 12	(3)	233 ± 43	(3)
Moxestrol	12 ± 1	(9)	122 ± 11	(7)
Estradiol	100		100	
2-Methyl estradiol	41 ± 6	(5)	7.1 ± 1.3	(5)
RU 15864	36 ± 7	(3)	5.8	(2)
Estriol	15 ± 2	(4)	4.3 ± 0.5	(3)
RU 16117	13 ± 1	(15)	4.0 ± 0.5	(7)
RU 26143 (J 60)	12 ± 1	(4)	2.1 ± 0.5	(4)
RU 2504	5.9 ± 0.5	(4)	31	(2)
Nafoxidine	1.9 ± 0.2	(3)	0.2	(2)
Tamoxifen	0.7	(2)	0.3	(2)

RBA values were measured as described under Material and Methods after 2 hr incubation at 0°C or 5 hr at 25°C. The results are the means of two determinations differing by less than 10% or the means ± S.E.M. of the number of determinations indicated in brackets.

incubation time and temperature were highly uterotrophic, as active (e.g. RU 2504) or more active (e.g. moxestrol, RU 5444 and ethynyl estradiol) than estradiol. Compound C 7701 was slightly less active than estradiol. On the contrary, compounds with RBA values decreasing with incubation time and temperature were weakly uterotrophic (about 300 times less potent than estradiol) with shallow dose-response curves.

All the compounds with RBA values decreasing with incubation time and temperature inhibited the increase in uterine weight induced by estradiol (Fig. 4). The most active (2-methyl estradiol and RU 26143 (J 60)) had RBA values decreasing 7 to 10 times. Inhibition by estradiol and RU 16117 was not dose-dependent probably because the uterotrophic activity of the higher doses prevailed upon their anti-uterotrophic activity.

II. Compounds that do not interact with the estrogenreceptor
Figure 5 lists a series of compounds, which do not normally compete for binding to the cytosolic estrogen receptor (Raynaud *et al.*, 1979), but which all interact with the progestin receptor of estrogen-primed rabbit uterus and/or with the androgen receptor of castrated rat

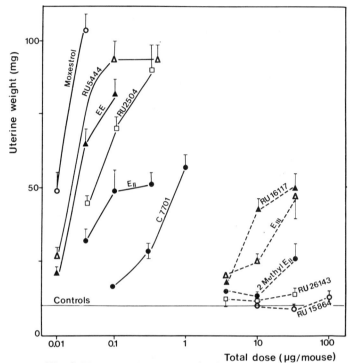

Fig. 3: Uterotrophic activity (s.c.) in the mouse

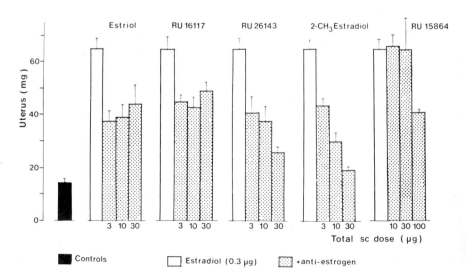

Fig. 4: Anti-uterotrophic activity (s.c.) in the mouse

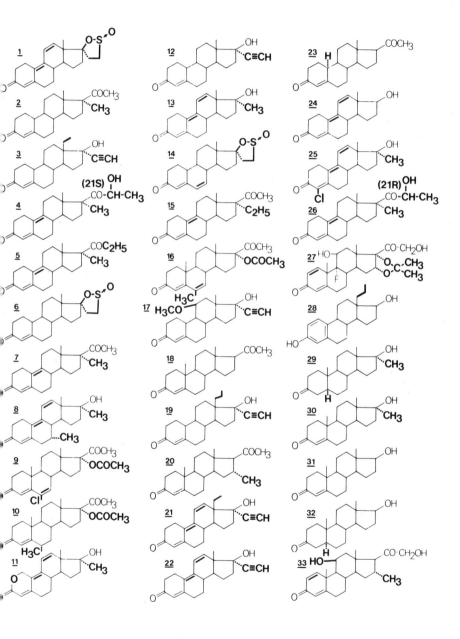

Fig. 5: Test-steroids

TABLE IV
Relative binding affinities for the progestin receptor
(RBA-Rp) in rabbit uterus and the androgen receptor
(RBA-R$_A$) in rat prostate.

		RBA-R$_p$ 24 hr 0°C		RBA-R$_A$ 2 hr 0°C	
1	(RU 25051)	869 ± 297	(4)	14 ± 1	(3)
2	(RU 3510)	916 ± 95	(4)	5.5 ± 1.6	(3)
3	Norgestrel	907 ± 184	(4)	87 ± 23	(5)
4	(RU 27987)	657 ± 33	(4)	2.4 ± 0.4	(3)
5	Promegestone	533 ± 40	(>90)	1.4 ± 0.4	(5)
6	(RU 22779)	337 ± 99	(4)	3.5 ± 1.5	(4)
7	Demegestone	420 ± 59	(4)	1.1 ± 0.4	(3)
8	(RU 2420)	330 ± 15	(3)	180 ± 23	(33)
9	Chlormadinone acetate	321 ± 35	(3)	20 ± 4	(3)
10	Medroxyprogesterone acetate	306 ± 25	(3)	51 ± 7	(4)
11	(RU 2999)	303 ± 24	(5)	158 ± 14	(3)
12	Norethindrone	263 ± 10	(3)	43 ± 3	(3)
13	Metribolone	191 ± 28	(3)	203 ± 5	(>50)
14	(RU 22761)	179 ± 6	(3)	<0.1	(2)
15	(RU 15182)	151 ± 31	(3)	0.45	(2)
16	Megestrol acetate	118 ± 10	(3)	19 ± 4	(4)
17	(RU 4843)	102 ± 14	(4)	2.8	(2)
18	Progesterone	100		5.5 ± 0.6	(3)
19	(RU 1364)	84 ± 3	(4)	44 ± 3	(3)
20	(RU 25845)	62 ± 9	(6)	1.0 ± 0.3	(5)
21	Gestrinone	48 ± 8	(8)	83 ± 3	(4)
22	Norgestrienone	47 ± 12	(5)	71 ± 13	(4)
23	(RU 18964)	40 ± 4	(3)	1.4	(2)
24	Trenbolone	16 ± 2	(3)	189 ± 24	(4)
25	(RU 2284)	15 ± 2	(3)	146 ± 8	(3)
26	(RU 27988)	13 ± 3	(4)	0.6 ± 0.2	(4)
27	Triamcinolone acetonide	12 ± 1	(3)	<0.1	(2)
28	(RU 1285)	2.7 ± 0.2	(3)	108 ± 23	(3)
29	Methylandrostanolone	2.4 ± 0.3	(4)	106 ± 19	(3)
30	Methyltestosterone	1.7	(2)	112 ± 7	(3)
31	Testosterone	1.1 ± 0.3	(3)	100	
32	5α-Dihydrotestosterone	0.9	(2)	120 ± 3	(10)
33	(RU 1178)	0.7 ± 0.1	(4)	0.2	(2)

RBA values were measured as described under Material and Methods after 24 hr incubation at 0°C (RBA-Rp) or 2 hr at 0°C (RBA-R$_A$). The results are expressed as in Table III.

prostate (Table IV). We have evaluated the anti-estrogenic activity of these compounds by measuring their ability to inhibit estrogen receptor replenishment (Fig. 6a) and the estradiol-induced increase in uterine wet weight (Fig. 6b) after a single s.c. injection. Since in each

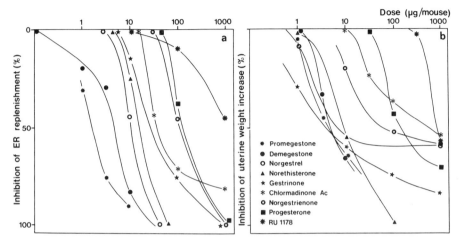

Fig. 6: Dose response curves (s.c.) in the mouse uterus. a) Inhibition of estrogen receptor replenishment, b) Inhibition of the estradiol-induced uterine weight increase. Estrogen-primed castrated mice were treated s.c. with estradiol (1 µg) alone or with estradiol plus various doses of test-steroids. Uterine weight and the uterine concentration of cytosolic estrogen receptor were determined as described under Material and Methods.

case inhibition was dose dependent and the inhibition curves were parallel, the anti-estrogenic activity of the test-compounds was compared by determining graphically the dose (ID_{50}) inhibiting the effect of estradiol by 50%. As shown in Fig. 7, there was a good linear correlation (r = 0.92) between the doses required to inhibit estrogen receptor replenishment and the estradiol-induced increase in uterine wet weight for compounds with low affinity for the androgen receptor (dots), but this correlation became somewhat poorer (r = 0.72) when the affinity for the androgen receptor increased (circles and stars). For compounds with low affinity for the androgen receptor (dots), there was a good correlation between binding to the progestin receptor and anti-uterotrophic activity (Fig. 8a) or inhibition of estrogen receptor replenishment (Fig. 8b) (r = 0.79 and 0.86 respectively). The higher the RBA value for progestin receptor binding, the greater the anti-estrogenic activity. If compounds with moderate affinity for the androgen receptor (circles) were included, the correlation between inhibition of replenishment and progestin binding (Fig. 8b) was not greatly modified (r = 0.82), but that between anti-uterotrophic activity and progestin binding (Fig. 8a)

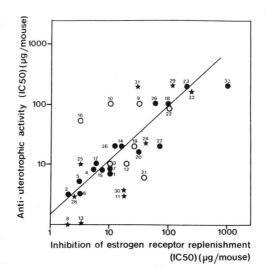

Fig. 7: Correlation between inhibition of the estradiolinduced uterine weight increase and inhibition of estrogen receptor replenishment. Compounds have been classified into 3 categories according to the RBA of their interaction with the androgen receptor. ● RBA-R$_A$ ⩽ 10, ○ 10 < RBA-R$_A$ < 100, * RBA-R$_A$ ⩾ 100.

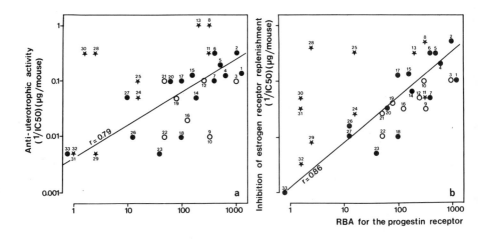

Fig. 8: Correlation between inhibition of the estradiolinduced uterine weight increase (a) or inhibition of estrogen receptor replenishment (b) and RBA's for the progestin receptor. ● RBA-R$_A$ ⩽ 10, ○ 10 < RBA-R$_A$ < 100, * RBA-R$_A$ ⩾ 100.

became poor (r = 0.62). If compounds with high affinity for the androgen receptor (stars) were included both correlations were extremely poor (r = 0.48 and 0.67, respectively).

Discussion

Anti-estrogen acting at the target organ level can be classified into at least two main categories, on the one hand, those that bind to the cytosolic estrogen receptor (like estriol, tamoxifen, dimethylstilbestrol or RU 16117) and that can be selected on the basis of their relative binding affinities (RBA's) for the estrogen receptor and, on the other hand, those that do not bind to the cytosolic estrogen receptor but interact with the progestin receptor. Since anti-uterotrophic activity is correlated with progestin receptor binding when androgen binding is weak, it is possible to screen for these latter compounds by measuring RBA values for the progestin receptor.

For anti-estrogenic activity, compounds belonging to the first category must not only inhibit estradiol binding to its receptor, but must themselves be weak estrogens unable to maintain, at low doses, a high nuclear estrogen-receptor concentration for the time normally required for a full estrogenic response (Anderson *et al.*, 1972 & 1975; Clark *et al.*, 1977). This could even apply to tamoxifen and nafoxidine in spite of the prolonged nuclear retention of the estrogen-receptor complex observed (Clark *et al.*, 1973; Jordan *et al.*, 1977) and which can be explained by continuous reloading of the receptor by the high doses injected (Bouton *et al.*, 1979; Chamness *et al.*, 1979). An analogous phenomenon occurs after injection of high RU 16117 doses (Bouton *et al.*, 1979).

Nuclear estrogen receptor retention depends upon the concentration of nuclear estrogen receptor and upon the dissociation rate of the nuclear complex. Since, as shown previously, the nuclear concentration of estrogen receptor depends upon the kinetics of the interaction with the cytosolic receptor (Bouton *et al.*, 1977) and since, as shown above, the nuclear complex retains the general properties of the cytosolic complex (i.e. a rapidly dissociating cytosolic complex gives rise to a rapidly dissociating nuclear complex), the nuclear concentration and retention of the estrogen-receptor complex must be directly related to the kinetic parameters of the interaction with the cytosolic estrogen receptor.

Thus, anti-estrogenic activity is promoted when the dissociation rate of the nuclear and, *a fortiori*, cytosolic complex is fast. All the anti-estrogens belonging to this category had this property in common (Bouton *et al.*, 1979; Capony *et al.*, 1977 & 1978; Katzenellenbogen *et al.*, 1978). It should therefore be possible to screen for potential antiestrogens by assessing interaction kinetics either directly or from RBA's measured under two sets of incubation conditions chosen in relation to the interaction kinetics of estradiol with its own receptor (Bouton et al., 1978). A compound with an RBA value decreasing with increasing incubation time and temperature will be a potential anti-hormone, a conclusion also valid for other steroid hormone classes (Bouton et al., 1978; Raynaud 1978 & 1979).

In contrast, compounds which after long incubation times have higher RBA values than after short incubation times will be potent agonists. Since there is a good correlation between anti-uterotrophic activity and binding to the progestin receptor, a compound with an RBA value for the progestin receptor increasing with incubation time will also be a potent anti-estrogen.

The anti-estrogenic activity of progesterone has been attributed to its inhibition of estrogen receptor replenishment rendering the uterus insensitive to subsequent estradiol injections (Bhakoo et al., 1977; Clark et al., 1977). However, our experiments do not entirely support this view since an anti-uterotrophic effect was observed after just a single injection before any specific effect on replenishment could take place, just as IP synthesis is inhibited after a single injection (Bhakoo et al., 1977). On the other hand, this anti-estrogenic activity could be due to inhibition of the binding of the nuclear estrogen receptor complex to the nuclear acceptor sites (Clark et al., 1977). In vivo, chlormadinone acetate inhibits nuclear uptake of tritiated estradiol, this effect being most marked 6 hr after injection, i.e. at a time when only nuclear acceptor sites are occupied by the nuclear estrogen receptor complex (Rosner et al., 1972).

Dihydrotestosterone and testosterone also have anti-estrogenic properties (Capony et al., 1978). They are able to compete with estradiol for estrogen-specific cytosolic binding sites in vitro under conditions which suggest that they form fast dissociating receptor complexes (Carcia et al., 1977 & 1979;Rochefort et al., 1976; Watson et al., 1977) and this competition could account for their anti-estrogenic properties. Both compounds also inhibit the replenishment of the cytosolic estrogen receptor, but, in our experiments, there was no correlation between anti-estrogenic acitivity and binding to the androgen receptor.

In conclusion, binding to the cytosolic estrogen and progestin receptors can be used to gauge potential anti-estrogenicity. Since the majority of hormone-dependent tumors contain both estrogen and progestin receptors (McGuire et al., 1977), either "pure" anti-estrogens or progestins could constitute appropriate forms of therapy, in particular those progestins that do not bind to the androgen receptor and are therefore devoid of androgenic side effects.

Acknowledgements

We wish to thank Professor J. Jacques and Dr. J. F. Miquel for kindly supplying us with some of the test-compounds, C. Pronin for her helpful collaboration and D. Gofflo for technical assistance.

References

Anderson, J. N., Clark, J. H. and Peck, E. J., JR. (1972). The relationship between nuclear receptor estrogen binding and uterotrophic responses. *Biochem. Biophys. Res. Comm.*, **48**, 1460-1468.

Anderson, J. N., Peck, E. J., JR. and Clark, J. H. (1975). Estrogen-induced uterine responses and growth : relationship to receptor estrogen binding by uterine nuclei. *Endocrinology*, **96**, 160-167.

Bhakoo, H. S. and Katzenellenbogen, B. S. (1977). Progesterone antagonism of estradiol-stimulated uterine "induced protein" synthesis. *Mol. Cell. Endocr.*, **8**, 105-120, 1977.

Bhakoo, H. S. and Katzenellenbogen, B. S. (1977). Progesterone modulation of estrogen-stimulated uterine biosynthetic events and estrogen receptor levels. *Mol. Cell. Endocr.*, **8**, 121-134.

Black, L. J. and Kraay, R. J. (1973). Evaluation of two types of estrogen inhibition with regard to effects on uptake and binding of (3H)-estradiol in the uterus. *J. Ster. Biochem.*, **4**, 467-475.

Bouton, M. M., Bonne, C. and Raynaud, J. P. (1978). "*In Vitro*" screening for anti-hormones. *J. Ster. Biochem.*, **9**, 836, 1978.

Bouton, M. M. and Raynaud, J. P. (1978). The relevance of kinetic parameters in the determination of specific binding to the estrogen receptor. *J. Ster. Biochem.*, **9**, 9-15, 1978.

Bouton, M. M. and Raynaud, J. P. (1977). Impaired nuclear translocation and regulation : a possible explanation of anti-estrogenic activity. *In: Research on steroids, vol* 7, (Vermeulen A., Klopper A., Sciarra F., Jungblut P. and Lerner L., eds), Elsevier, North-Holland Biomedical Press, pp. 127-136.

Bouton, M. M. and Raynaud, J. P. (1979). The relevance of interaction kinetics in determining biological response. *Endocrinology*, **105**, 509-515.

Capony, F. and Rochefort, H. (1977). *In vitro* and *in vivo* interactions of (3H) dimethylstilbestrol with the estrogen receptor. *Mol. Cell. Endocrinol.*, **8**, 47-64.

Capony, F. and Rochefort, H.(1978). High affinity binding of the anti-estrogen (3H) tamoxifen to the 8S estradiol receptor. *Mol. Cell. Endocrinol.*, **11**, 181-198.

Chamness, G. C. and Bromley, J. M. (1979). Rapid turnover of receptor-anti-estrogen complexes in nuclei. *In: Abstracts, The Endocri Society, June 1979*, p. 275 no 810.

Chauveau, J., Moule, Y. and Rouiller, CH. (1956). Isolation of pure and un-altered liver nuclei, morphology and biochemical compositon. *Exp. Cell Res.*, **11**, 317-321.

Clark, J. H., Anderson, J. N. and Peck, E. J. JR. (1973). Estrogen receptor anti-estrogen complex: A typical binding by uterine nuclei and effects on uterine growth. *Steroids*, **22**, 707-718.

Clark, J. H., Hsueh, A. J. W. and Peck, E. J. JR. (1977). Regulation of estrogen receptor replenishment by progesterone. *Ann. N. Y. Acad. Sci. (U.S.A.)*, **286**, 161-179.

Clark, J. H., Paszko, Z. and Peck, E. J. JR. (1977). Nuclear binding and retention of the receptor estrogen complex: relation to the agonistic and antagonistic properties of estriol. *Endocrinology*, **100**, 91-96.

Desombre, E. R. and Arbogast, L. Y. (1974). Effect of the antiestrogen CI628 on the growth of rat mammary tumors. *Cancer. Res.*, **34**, 1971-1976.

DI Carlo, F., Conti, G. and Reboani, C. (1978). Interference of gestagens and androgens with rat uterine oestrogen receptors. *J. Endocr.*, **77**, 49-55.

Emmens, C. W. and Miller, B. G. (1969). Estrogen, proestrogens and anti-estrogens. *Steroids*, **13**, 725-730.

Garcia, M. and Rochefort, H. (1977). Androgens on the estrogen receptor. II - Correlation between nuclear translocation and uterine protein synthesis. *Steroids*, **29**, 111-126.

Garcia, M. and Rochefort, H. (1979). Evidence and characterization of the binding of two 3H-labeled androgens to the estrogen receptor. *Endocrinology*, **104**, 1797-1804.

Jordan, V. C. (1976). Effect of Tamoxifen (ICI 46,474) on initiation and growth of DMBA-induced rat mammary carcinomata. *Europ. J. Cancer*, **12**, 419-424.

Jordan, V. C., Dix, C. J., Rowsby, L. and Prestwich, G. (1977). Studies on the mechanism of action of the nonsteroidal antioestrogen tamoxifen (I.C.I. 46, 474) in the rat. *Mol. Cell. Endocr.*, **7**, 177-192.

Katzenellenbogen, B. S., Katzenellenbogen, J. A., Ferguson, E. R. and Krauthammer, N. (1978). Anti-estrogen interaction with uterine estrogen receptors. *J. Biol. Chem.*, **253**, 697-707.

Kelly, P. A., Asselin, J., Labrie, F. and Raynaud, J. P. (1977). Regulation of hormone receptor levels and growth of DMBA-induced mammary tumors by RU 16117 and other steroids in the rat. *In: Progesterone Receptors in Normal and Neoplastic Tissue*, (McGuire W. L., Raynaud J. P. and Baulieu E. E., eds), Raven Press, New York, pp. 85-101.

Korenman, S. G. (1970). Relation between estrogen inhibitory activity and binding to cytosol of rabbit and human uterus. *Endocrinology*, **87**, 1119-1123.

Lerner L. J. (1964). Hormone antagonists: Inhibitors of specific activities of estrogen and androgen. *Rec. Progr. Horm. Res.*, **20**, 435-490.

McGuire, W. L., Raynaud, J. P. and Baulieu, E. E. (Eds.) (1977). Progesterone Receptors in Normal and Neoplastic Tissues, *Prog. Cancer Res. Ther., vol.* **4**,. Raven Press, New York.

Nicholson, R. I. and Golder, M. P. (1975). Effect of synthetic anti-estrogens on the growth and biochemistry of rat mammary tumors. *Eur. J. Cancer*, **11**, 571-579.

Raynaud, J. P. (1978). The mechanism of action of anti-hormones. *In: Advances in Pharmacology and Therapeutics*, vol. **1**, Receptors, (Jacob J., ed), Pergamon Press, Oxford, pp. 259-278.

Raynaud, J. P. and Bercovici, J. P. (1979). Introduction à la pharmacologie des progestatifs de synthèse. *Ann. Endocrinol. (Paris)*, **40**, 300-320.

Raynaud, J. P., Bonne, C., Bouton, M. M., Lagace, L. and Labrie, F. (1979). Action of a non-steroid anti-androgen, RU 23908, in peripheral and central tissues. *J. Ster. Biochem.*, **11**, 93-99.

Raynaud, J. P., Martin, P., Bouton, M. M. and Ojasoo, T. (1978). 11β-Methoxy-17-ethynyl-1,3,5(10)-estratriene-3,17b-diol (Moxestrol), a tag for estrogen receptor-binding sites in human tissues. *Cancer. Res.*, **38**, 3044-3050.

Raynaud, J. P., Ojasoo, T., Bouton, M. M. and Philibert, D. (1979). Receptor binding as a tool in the development of new bioactive steroids. *In: Drug Design*, vol. **VIII**, (Ariens E. J., ed), Academic Press, New York, pp. 170-214.

Rochefort, H. and Garcia, M. (1976). Androgen on the estrogen receptor. I - Binding and *in vivo* nuclear translocation. *Steroids*, **28**, 549-560.

Rosner, J. M., Macome, J. C., Denari, J. H. and De Carli, D. N. (1972). Antioestrogenic action of chlormadinone acetate. *Acta Endocrinol.*, **69**, 403-409.

Terenius, L. (1971). Antioestrogens and breast cancer. *Eur. J. Cancer*, **7**, 57-64.

Watson, G. H., Korach, K. S. and Muldoon, T. G. (1977). Obstruction of estrogen-receptor complex formation. Further analysis of the nature and steroidal specificity of the effect. *Endocrinology*, **101**, 1733-1743.

Discussion

Hospital: X Ray analysis of a molecule gives the precise description of its conformation and interactions. Though the study is made in the crystal the conformation is the most probable and the quality and intensity of the observed interactions have a good probability of being found when the molecule is fixed on its receptor. In these conditions it is best to use X ray results to try to establish a structure-affinity relationship. The affinity of a substrate for a receptor depends for a great part on the geometrical aspect of the interactions. X ray analysis have been made for many molecules belonging to different chemical families and showing a good affinity for the cyto-

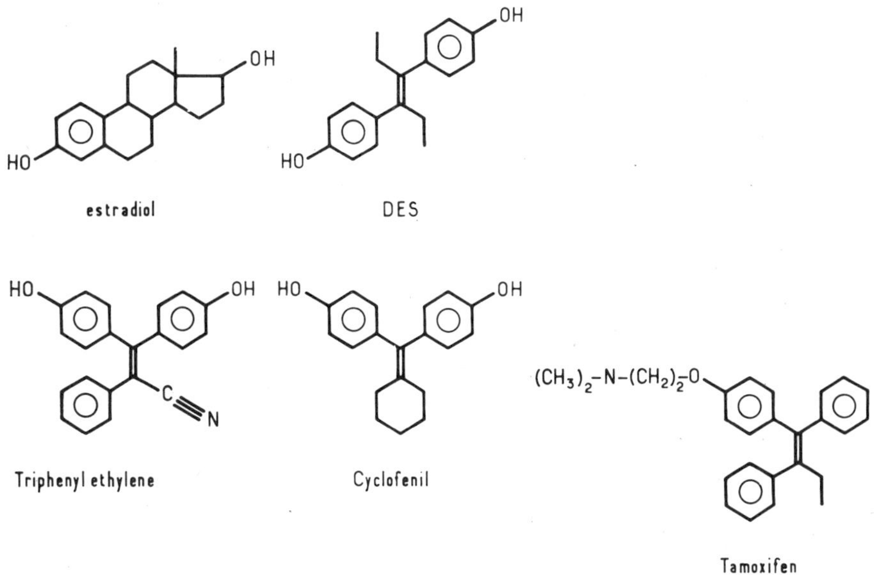

Fig. 1: Some estrogenic compounds studied by x ray analysis (diéthylstilbestrol = DES).

solic uterin receptor.

Estradiol, the natural hormone, is sufficiently undeformable to be the reference for the geometrical superposition of the molecular conformation of different molecules. We have found two different conformations for diethylstilbestrol (parallel or non parallel phenolic rings) depending on whether the crystallization was done from hydrophobic or hydrophilic solutions (Busetta *et al.*, 1973). We have chosen the dissymetrical conformation showing crossed and non parallel phenolic rings as the "active" form after the comparison with estradiol geometry as well as for some other biochemical and biological reasons. X ray analysis of some triphenyl ethylene derivatives has shown the same "active" conformation when the two aromatic groups are trans to the double bond. The superposition (Fig. 2) of molecules of estradiol, diethylstilbestrol and triphenyl ethylene derivatives shows the general shape necessary for binding to the receptor. The comparison of modifications made to the general skeleton by the addition of different side groups and the values of the affinity coefficients suggest some modifications able to increase or diminish the affinity constant. We have then the possibility of proposing molecules which will probably be very good estrogens. Such predictions are of little therapeutic interest but that is not the case for the prediction of new antiestrogens. An antiestrogen could be a molecule having strong affinity for the estrogenic receptor but being a bad transmitter of the information necessary to start the processes characteristic of the activity.

We have two possibilities to reach this goal: examination of geometrical aspects or examination of the kinetics of the formation of substrate-receptor complexes.

X ray crystallography could make a contribution to the first aspect

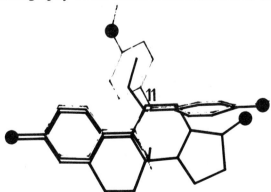

Fig. 2: Superposition of estradiol, DES and triphenylethylene derivative

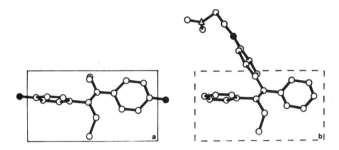

Fig. 3: Crystal Structure of DES (a) and tamoxifene (b)

of the problem. The comparison of the conformation of the "estrogenic skeleton" already described and the conformation of an antiestrogenic molecule used in therapeutics could suggest structure modifications necessary for antiestrogenic properties. If we add to the previous figure the structure (Fig. 3) of tamoxifene the importance of position 11 of the estradiol is evident in determining the degree of activity of the steroid (Hospital *et al.*, 1975; Precigouc, 1978).

The purpose of crystallography is to provide the structural requirements for estrogenic compounds to bind to the receptor and to clarify which substitutions can be used for anti-estrogenic activity. It remains for the chemist to use this information in the synthesis of related molecules, and for the biologists to determine the physiological activity and side effects. It is only after all this work has been done that the hypothesis of the crystallographer can be confirmed.

Katzenellenbogen: Many anti-estrogens have triarylethylene structures. Potentially there are two ways you can superimpose these on estradiol: one with the third phenyl group going off and the other with the phenyl group going down. Do you have any feeling which one of these is the way these compounds are bound to the receptor?

Hospital: I think the two conformations are possible: one with the aryl group hanging out at position 11 and one with the aryl group on position 7. We have synthesized molecules for affinity chromatography, with attachment at positions 7 and 11. For affinity chromatography position 7 seems better. Although for the model (triarylethylene superimposed on estradiol), I prefer the conformation with an aryl group at position 11 because for a triarylethylene the substitution in the direction of the D-ring is better.

Hochberg: I noticed that one of your compounds, I think it was the

12-β-methyl compound, was extremely active.

Hospital: I have just obtained the result of the affinity but we haven't studied the structure.

Reference

Busetta, B., Courseille, C., & Hospital, M. (1973). *Acta Cryst.*, **B29**, 2456-2462.
Hospital, M. Busetta, B., Courseille, C., & Precigoux G. (1975). *J. of Steroid Biochem.*, **6**, 221-225.
Precigoux, G., (1978). Thèse doctorat ès Sciences - Université de Bordeaux I (France).

COVALENT BINDING OF ESTROGEN DERIVATIVES TO α-FETOPROTEIN

G. VAN BINST, G. LAUS, M. VAN GENECHTEN
A. BAREL, V. VERSEE, R. ZEEUWS

V.U.B., Brussels, Belgium

Synthesis

We have been interested for some time in the interaction of steroid analogs and derivatives with binding proteins or receptors. First attempts were made by nuclear magnetic resonance but the concentration range of this method is far away from the physiological conditions.

During the last years we focussed our attention on the photolabeling techniques of steroids, to identify the amino-acids at the binding site of the binding proteins. This can be done after total hydrolysis of the complex by mass spectrometry and nuclear magnetic resonance on the partially hydrolysed labeled peptides.

The following steroid derivatives were synthesized: 3-azidohexestrol (I), 3,3'-diazidohexestrol (II), 2-azidoestrone (III), 4-azidoestrone (IV), 2-azidoestradiol (V), 4-azidoestradiol (VI), estradiol-17β-diazoacetate (VII) and 11-α-diazoacetyloxyestrone (VIII) (Fig. 2). We are grateful to Dr. Zeelen (Organon Scientific Development Group) for the supply of 11-α-hydroxyestrone.

The synthesis of these compounds has been achieved according to known procedures (1) which occasionally were modified (Fig. 3, 4).

We have tried to synthesize the estradiol derivatives by direct nitration of the parent steroid. However since we didn't obtain reasonable yields we had to go back to the reduction of the corresponding aminoestrone to estradiol.

Concerning 11-α-diazoacetyloxyestrone (VIII), all attempts to perform a direct formation of the diazoacetate failed and gave only the

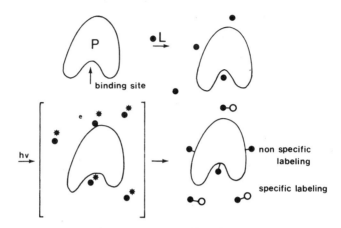

O = solvent or scavenger
Fig. 1: Principle of photoaffinity labeling

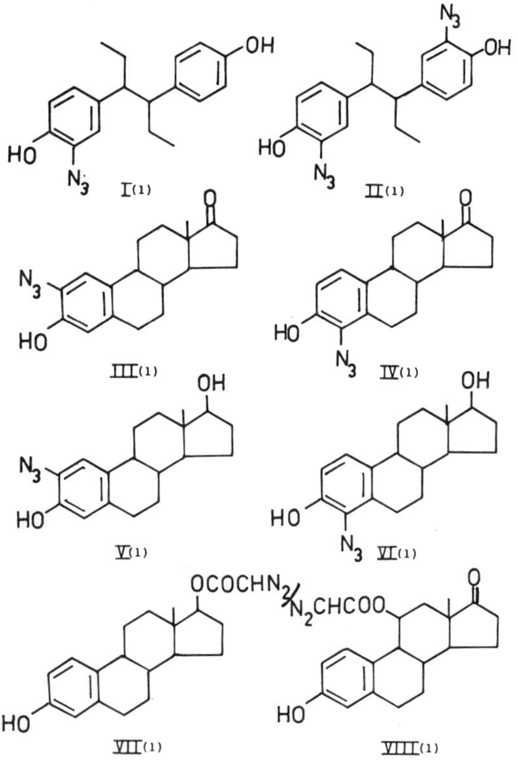

Fig. 2: Photoaffinity labels

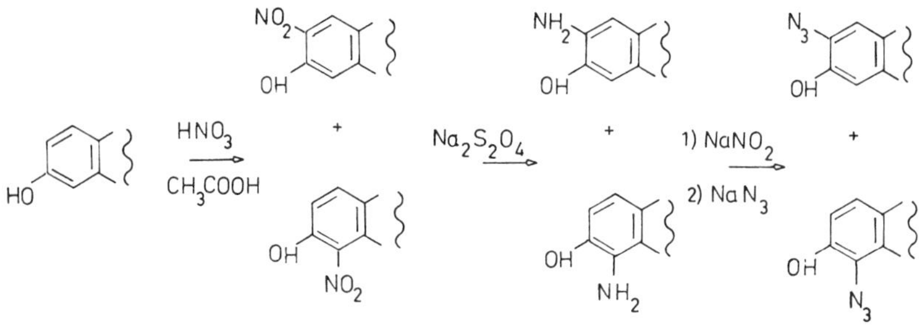

Fig. 3: General Procedures (1)

starting product. Work is in progress to protect the 3-OH position by acetylation with 3-acetyl-1,5,5-trimethylhydantoin prior to the reaction with the acid chloride of glyoxilic acid tosylhydrazone.

Photochemical behaviour

In order to evaluate the reactivity of the photolabels, reaction velocity and completeness, 4-azidoestron and 17β-estradiol diazoacetate were irradiated at 254 nm and 315 nm in a tetrahydrofurane solution. After 15 min. irradiation of a 80 mg solution, the azido- or $-C=N^{\oplus}=N^{\ominus}$ peak disappears in the I.R.-spectrum. The resulting products were analysed by mass-spectrometry and the structure of the C-H insertion products was determined. At 254 nm, some ring cleavage products of the bound tetrahydrofurane ring appear but at 315 nm only pure C-H insertion products are detected. Insertion occurs at the 2 position of tetrahydrofuran as well as in the 3 position (Fig. 5). Analogous experiments performed in methanol gave predominantly the starting products.

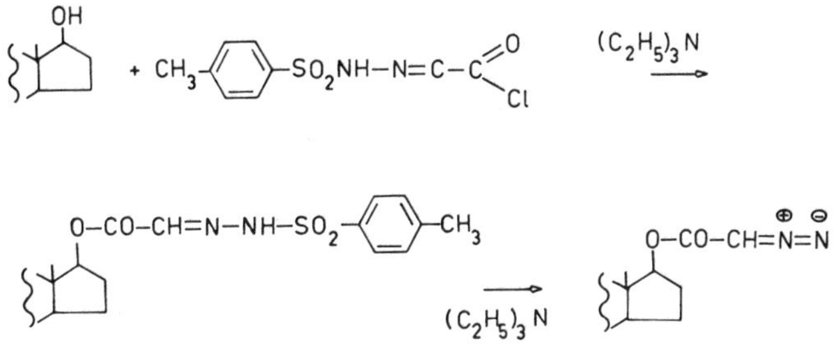

Fig. 4: General Procedures (2)

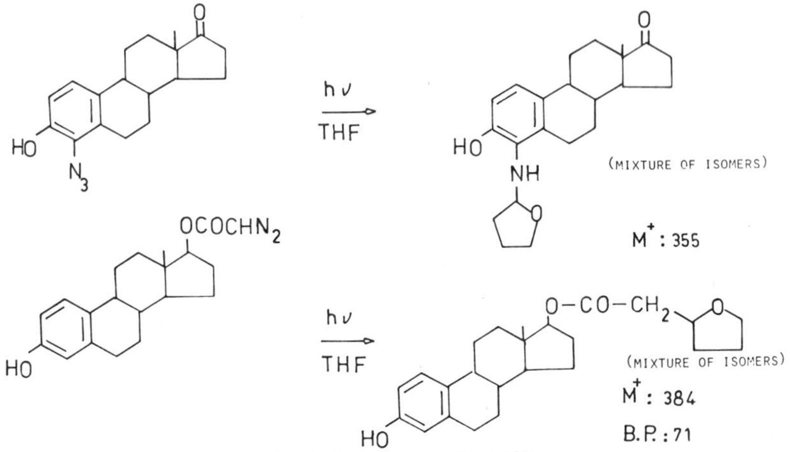

Fig. 5: Reaction with THF

Binding studies

In order to compare the modified substrates with the original steroids, binding studies were carried out with α-feto-protein (AFP). The experiments on the binding of estradiol or other ligands to α-feto-protein were carried out by the Sephadex G25 technique described by Pearlmann and Crépy (1967) and Goertz et al., (1973).

The method can be compared with an equilibrium dialysis: protein (P) and radiolabeled steroid bound to the protein (S_b), are excluded by the dextrangel (Sephadex G25) and remain in the external phase. The unbound steroid (S_u), partitions freely between the external and internal phase of the dextran.

The binding data are analysed according to Scatchard (1949)

$$\frac{S_b}{S_u} = P \cdot n - K_a \cdot S_b$$

Displacement studies

To study the interactions of unlabeled steroids with α-fetoprotein, displacement experiments of bound radiolabeled estradiol were carried out.

A constant amount of (^{3}H) estradiol was added to each tube. Various quantities of unlabeled steroids were added to displace the bound (^{3}H) estradiol. From the radioactivity in the external volume, the amount of labeled estradiol bound to the α-fetoprotein can be calculated. The residual binding was plotted against the total amount of added ligand.

The equilibrium relationship between (^{3}H) estradiol and the ligand for a single binding site is given by a simple equation.

$$\left(\frac{S_u}{S_b}\right)_A = \frac{K_{ES}}{K_A} \left(\frac{S_u}{S_b}\right)_{ES}$$

where S_u = free, S_b = bound
K = association constant.
The subscripts A and ES refer to ligand and estradiol, respectively. The ratio of the instrinsic association constants $\dfrac{K_{ES}}{K_A}$ or $\dfrac{K_A}{K_{ES}}$ may be considered as an index of competition. If K_{ES} is known the value of K_A can be readily calculated from a simple linear plot. In this plot $\left(\dfrac{S_u}{S_b}\right)_A$ is plotted against $\left(\dfrac{S_u}{S_b}\right)_{ES}$. (Versée and Barel, 1978).
From Table I, it is apparent that most of the photolabeling reagents bind fairly well with constants in the 10^6 range and that 4-azido-estrone has the highest binding constant.

Purification of α-fetoprotein (rat)

At the appropriate gestational age (15-19 days), amniotic fluid and fetal plasma were collected from Wistar rat fetuses. The purification procedure has been described previously by Cittanova *et al.,* (1974) and Kerckaert *et al.,* (1975). Briefly the first purification step consists of elimination of hemoglobin by batchwise adsorption on CM-cellulose (carboxy-methyl-cellulose) in 0.01 M potassium phosphate buffer, pH 6.0. The second purification step is achieved by passage through a blue Sepharose Cl-6B column in order to remove selectively most of the albumin fraction. The third purification step involves a preparative polyacrylamide slab-gel electrophoresis. Examination of preparations of α-fetoprotein on analytical polyacrylamide gel electrophoresis revealed a preparation free of contaminating proteins such as albumin, transferrin and globulins. The analytical acrylamide-gel electrophoresis revealed the typical microheterogeneity of this protein: two slow moving bands and one fast moving band.

Defatting of α-fetoprotein

Since human α-fetoprotein contains fatty acids (Parmelee *et al.,* 1978), the defatting of rat α-fetoprotein was routinely carried out. This step involves the passage through a small column containing an anion exchanger AG-1-X8. Elution was carried out with acetic acid 0.1 M, pH 2.9. Immediately after passage through the column, the AFP containing fractions were neutralized, dialysed and lyophilized.

Photoaffinity labeling; Photoinactivation of α-fetoprotein

The sample tubes contained usually in a total volume of 3 ml TRIS-EDTA buffer, pH 7.4, about 5 mg of pure defatted α-fetoprotein (70 nmoles). This amount of AFP was incubated with a small volume (10 μl) of photoaffinity label (20 to 700 nmoles) freshly dissolved in tetrahydrofuran. All the aqueous solutions were saturated with nitrogen. Photolyses were carried out at a wavelength higher than 315 nm for 15 minutes at a temperature of 2-8° C. Blank experiments were carried out in the presence of tetrahydrofuran without the photoaffinity label. The non-covalently bound affinity label was removed from the protein after the irradiation, by extensive dialysis in the cold (4°C) (48 hours against the same buffer, then against potassium-phosphate buffer at pH 8.5). The residual binding capacity of the chemically modified protein towards (^{3}H) estradiol was measured using the Sephadex gel binding assay. The results of these experiments are expressed as Association constants and molar concentrations of bindings sites. The concentration of protein was determined at 280 nm or by a color reaction (Folin).

The results are summarized in Table II.

Table II

Experimental Condition	Molar ratio Label/Protein	N	K 10^7	% label
Blanco (1)	-	0.78	2.3	-
	0.3	0.64	2.6	12
	3.0	0.54	2.2	30
(2)	10	0.48	1.7	36
Repetitive irradiation (3) (3x)	10	0.48	1.4	36

These results show a significant lowering of the stoichiometry which means that at least 36% of the photoaffinity label is bound irreversibly to the protein at the binding site. The non significant variations of K indicate only a small denaturation of the protein during the experiment.

Further experiments are in progress with irradiation of AFP protected by bound estradiol in the presence of photoaffinity label compounds and also with radiolabeled material to determine the total amount of specifically bound material.

The initial analyses were done on the hydrolysates of the mixture of photolabeled AFP and AFP. These hydrolysates were purified by reversed phase (C18) HPLC, the covalently labeled amino acids are retained on the column. The MS analysis of this retained fraction is in progress.

To determine the structure of the binding site, two major strategies will be followed in the future:

1. separation of AFP, from the labeled AFP by affinity chromatography, degradation by hydrolysis of the bound AFP, separation of the labeled amino acids and peptides by HPLC, identification of the fragments by mass spectrometry.
2. direct hydrolysis of the mixture of labeled and unlabeled AFP, separation of the labeled fragments by an AFP-affinity column followed by HPLC and MS.

References

Cittanova, N., Grigorova, A., Benassayag, C., Munez, E. and Jayle, M. F. (1974), *FEBS Lett.* **41**, 21-24.

Goertz, G. R., Guérin, Crépy, O. C., Longchampt, J. E. and Jayle M. F. (1973), *Eur. J. Biochem.* **35**, 311-317.

Katzenellenbogen, J. A., Meyers, H. N., Johnson, H. J. Jr., (1973), *J. Org. Chem.* **38**, 3525.

Kerckaert, J. P., Bayard, B., Quief, S. and Biserte, G. (1975), *FEBS Lett.* **53**, 234-236.

Parmelee, D. C., Evenson, M. A. and Deutsch, H. F. (1978), *J. Biol. Chem.* **253**, 2114-2119.

Pearlman, W. H. and Crépy, O. (1967), *J. Biol. Chem.* **242**, 182-189.

Scatchard, G. (1949), *Ann. N. Y. Acad. Sci* **51**, 660-672.

Versée, V. and Barel, A. O., (1978), *FEBS Lett.* **96**, 155-158.

Versée, V., and Barel, A. O. (1978), *Biochem. J.,* **175**, 73-81.

Discussion

Sandberg: Why did you choose α-fetoprotein?

Van Binst: α-fetoprotein is a protein of the amniotic fluid which binds estrogens very well.

Sandberg: Not in the human.

Van Binst: We used rat α-fetoprotein.

Katzenellenbogen: In the table of percent inactivation which compound did you use?

Van Binst: It was the 4-azido derivative.

Katzenellenbogen: Do you have comparable data on the other photosensitive molecules?

Van Binst: No, we didn't try the others because the 4-azido derivative was the one with the highest binding constant.

Katzenellenbogen: We have also been interested in photoaffinity-labeling of α-fetoprotein. We studied 4-azidoestradiol and 16-diazoestradiol. Both compounds looked comparable in terms of their inactivation which is on the order of 15%. When we used the tritiated compound the 4-azido compound looked very poor, but the 16-diazo looked like a reasonable efficient photoaffinity-label.

Barel: The binding of steroids to the cellular receptors has predominantly been studied using radiolabeled hormones. Another possibility of investigation involves the use of fluorescent labeled steroids.

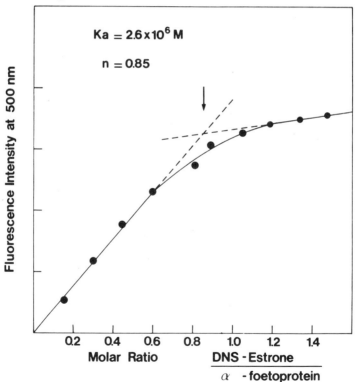

Fig. 1: Fluorimetric titration of defatted α-fetoprotein (7.1 μM) with DNS-estrone (from 1.1 to 10.5 μM) in 0.01 M-potassium phosphate buffer, pH 7.4.

The fluorescence properties of these probes are markedly changed when bound to a receptor or to a steroid binding protein. In this short report we present the synthesis of 3-0-dansyl estrone and its binding with α-fetoprotein. Estrone was mixed with dansyl chloride in a water/acetone basic solution (addition of NaHCO$_3$). The reaction mixture was extracted with ethyl acetate. DNS-estrone was further purified by HPLC. The homogeneity of our preparation was ascertained by mass spectrometry. The addition of α-fetoprotein to DNS-estrone produced an increase of fluorescence and a blue shift of the dye. The stoichiometry and association constant of the protein-dye complex were determined by fluorometric titration. α-Fetoprotein binds 0.85 mol of fluorescent label with an association constant of 2.6 x 10^6 M (Fig. 1). DNS-estrone binding to the protein was also confirmed by equilibrium gel filtration using a tritium labeled dye. Displacement experiments of bound DNS-estrone with linoleic acid and estradiol were carried out to determine whether these ligands

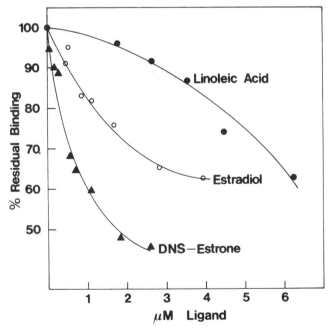

Fig. 2: Displacement of bound DNS-estrone with various ligands. The gel equilibration assay with Sephadex G-25 was used in 0.1 M- potassium phosphate buffer, ph 7.4 at 25°C. A constant concentration of [^{3}H] labeled DNS-estrone (45 nM) and α-fetoprotein (5.25 nM) was considered for each tube. Various amounts of the ligands were added as shown (from 90 - 6000 nM). The amount of labeled DNS-estrone bound to α-fetoprotein was calculated from the radioactivity of the external phase.

could compete for the binding site (Fig. 2). Both ligands were able to displace the bound dye, suggesting a competition for the steroid binding site. These data show the rather high affinity of this fluorescent steroid for a steroid binding and suggest its potential use for binding studies with cell receptor proteins.

PANEL DISCUSSION

Wittliff: What part of the molecule is really the best from the standpoint of attachment of a cytotoxic group?

Katzenellenbogen: I can speak about the non-steroidal compounds probably because this was the system with which we had most experience. We really made two types of derivatives; one was substituted in the aromatic ring adjacent to the phenolic hydroxyl and the other at the end of the hexane chain. It is interesting to think of these in terms of the corresponding positions in the steroidal compounds, to see some comparative feature between steroidal and non-steroidal estrogens. We found that the position ortho to the hydroxyl group in a compound such as hexestrol is reasonably tolerant to fairly large substitutions. The largest groups would have been iodine and azide but that is smaller than anything cytotoxic. I think Hans Hamacher has made some nitrogen mustards at this position. This position seems to be reasonably tolerant to substitution, particularly if you compare the corresponding 2- and 4-substituted estradiols, but one should realize that the hexestrol is a flexible symmetrical molecule. So that one is actually making two enantiomers which may present the groups in as many as four different positions at the receptor site. The derivatives we made at the end of the hexane chain, which might correspond to substitutions at 7α or 11β of estradiols which are fairly tolerant in the steroidal estrogens, seem to be positions with considerable bulk tolerance.

Hospital: I have several answers. It depends on what is the starting molecule (steroid or not). We have tried to make several substrates for affinity chromatography. It works if we put the long chain on the steroid molecule in the 7α positon or in the 17α position.

But when we tried to do the same with triphenylethylene the best position was not on the three arylic rings but on the part of the molecule corresponding to the 7-position of the steroid.

Hochberg: Dr. Katzenellenbogen I wonder whether you have tried to quantitate the uterine uptake. In the slide you showed of the various compounds that had merit factors, did you attempt to quantitate the uterine uptake and to correlate it with these merit factors?

Katzenellenbogen: We haven't done this extensively because we only made the table a short while ago and so we have not really done the appropriate biological studies to correlate with it. There is one bit of data which I think does fit in very nicely and I mentioned it very briefly. This concerns the relative potency of estradiol and estriol. It is very important what kind of biological response you choose because Clark has shown that the duration of receptor occupancy is very important, particularly long duration being required for a long term response. If you are comparing short term responses in terms of receptor translocation and you compare the potency of estradiol to the one of estriol in an *in vitro* system (this is the work of Anderson and Clark), there is a big difference in potency between estradiol and estriol. Estriol looks about 5% as potent as estradiol, which compares well with the ratio of the receptor affinities. If you do the translocation experiment *in vivo* where now you have albumin and all the non-specific binders competing for the binding of this ligand, they appear to be more or less equally active. According to my merit factor estimates, the merit factors of estradiol and estriol are much more comparable than are the receptor binding affinities. So I think that that example is consistent with the numbers. I would very much like to do the experiment with 6-oxo-estradiol which I would predict may be even more potent than estradiol.

Sandberg: It is not enough to know where to put the anti-tumor agent in the molecule. But once you get it into the cell it must come off. So now you are faced with two serious problems: where to put the agent to get it carried in and secondly it must come off.

Katzenellenbogen: I think that depends on the choice of the anti-tumor agent. If it is something that can react with DNA....

Sandberg: It will not react with DNA if it has this giant steroid attached to it.

Katzenellenbogen: Well that is just a question of access to DNA which is a separate issue.

Wittliff: We don't have a lot of data on this but by taking isolated chromatin or isolated DNA and letting it interact with estradiol-mustards, we found some evidence that it interacted directly with DNA, even when the steroid was apparently attached to the mustard.
So I am not convinced as yet that you have to hydrolyse the conjugate to do some damage to the nucleus.

Sandberg: If you are saying that you are producing the anti-tumor effect by affecting the estrogen receptor complex activity on the chromatin, you don't need the anti-tumor agent. The idea is to get the anti-tumor agent into the cell because the estrogen gets into the cell. Once it is in the cell you have to get it off so it acts as an anti-tumor agent.

Wittliff: But what we don't know is whether the estradiol-mustard or estracyt has its anti-tumor effect as the intact molecule.

Konives: There is a big difference in the alkylating properties of a nitrogen mustard group depending on whether the nitrogen is bound directly to for example, an aromatic ring or to a carbonyl function. In the first case the nitrogen is rather basic, enhancing the alkylating abilities of the β-chloroethyl group thus making this type of compound very reactive. In the second case the nitrogen is not basic at all and hydrolysis of the carbamate is necessary to get a mustard moiety with alkylating properties.

Katzenellenbogen: I once developed a terminology in which I used two terms to describe a steroid-receptor reagent: one in which the functional group is in an integral part of the steroid, the integrated reagents, as opposed to the conjugated reagents, where you just take a functional component and attach it to the ligand moiety. Another question which comes up: to what extent is the activity of the agent enhanced by its integration, its conjugation to the ligand. To what extent does it have to be hydrolyzed before it is active. In these terms we can at least discuss the issue more precisely.

Hochberg: Dr.Sandberg do you have reason to believe that if the estrogen moiety is still on the nitrogen mustard, it won't react with DNA?

Sandberg: Some of them won't, others will.

Hospital: Is it so important that the steroid used as a carrier has a good affinity for the receptor? Perhaps it is possible to increase the affinity of the steroid for the transporter and not for the receptor.

Katzenellenbogen: I would like to ask Dr. Wittliff to comment whether he thinks there is a difference between the transporter and the receptor.
There were some experiments that were done that suggest that there was a carrier mediated uptake system for estrogens in target tissues. But my impression is that it is no longer considered.

Wittliff: The receptor is the transporter in any cell system that I know of and I would like to hear if there is any disagreement with that general statement.

Katzenellenbogen: I think that we have to keep clearly in mind what we are trying to do. We are trying to use receptors to provide a mechanism for selective concentration in receptor containing cells. It then follows necessarily that the agent has to be a good binder for the receptor and has to be a selective binder, that's where the merit factor comes in. The drug must be able to bind to the receptor to a larger extent than to albumin. On the other hand, there are a lot of potentials for artefacts in work of this type and I think these have indeed appeared in the early literature on agents of this type.
Whenever you make a derivative, activity can go up or it can go down and selectivity can go up or it can go down. Just because it happens to be attached to an estrogen doesn't necessarily mean that because the activity of the derivative goes up, it is because it is interacting selectively with the receptor. It may be for a completely different reason. It may just be due to the duration of action or to a depot formation or something like that. This means that experiments that demonstrate enhanced selectivity or enhanced activity of steroid-cytotoxic conjugates have to be able to establish that the action is proceeding by a receptor mediated process. If you get a better agent just because it is more or less lipophilic that may be a beneficial thing to do, but this is not based on receptor interaction.

Hochberg: Dr. Katzenellenbogen do you mean that a compound could have a worse merit factor and still be better?

Katzenellenbogen: Yes, but not by a receptor mediated process.

Zeelen: I have a feeling that we are wrong in our way of looking at it and that we make one basic mistake. We want to make use of the possibility of the estradiol molecule binding to the receptor, to get the cytotoxic agent into the nucleus. We have to realize what happens. As soon as the complex binds it will be neatly surrounded by the receptor protein.

We have taken a reagent designed for interaction with RNA or DNA which we now have completely wrapped in a protein surrounding. This means that we have more or less inactivated it. I think that we have to compromise on the whole thing. We have to find just that sort of binding which would be sufficient to get the complex into the nucleus but on the other hand a binding that is not too strong so that the cytotoxic agent can come off.

Katzenellenbogen: If the conjugate has to act while it is bound to the receptor than you may need an arm to provide access to the DNA. I think Dr. Zeelen brought up an interesting concept that there is probably an optimal binding activity that will enable the compound to dissociate sufficiently from the receptor once it is in the nucleus, in order to reach DNA just by coming off the receptor. I want to raise an other point, that is, the receptor nuclear interaction is a dynamic one and if you just inject estradiol you see nuclear receptor levels go up and then they go down. What happens when they go down? Is the steroid being released in the nucleus or is the receptor coming back into the cytoplasm when the steroid is released. I think most people would say that whatever happens to the receptor-estrogen complex in the nucleus it is a mysterious phenomenon. It is probably going to release the free steroid in the nucleus and that is a process which may be of benefit in achieving selective cytotoxicity.

SYNTHESIS OF CYTOTOXIC ESTROGENS

ESTROGEN-CATHARANTHUS (VINCA) ALKALOID CONJUGATES

ROBERT P. BLICKENSTAFF, KOERT GERZON

Veterans Administration Medical Center, and Department of Biochemistry, and Department of Pharmacology, Indiana University School of Medicine, Indianapolis, Indiana, USA

Introduction

The preparation and biological activity of steroid-alkylating agent, steroid-nucleoside, and other steroid-antitumor agent conjugates has been reported in the period since World War II (Carroll *et al.*, 1972; Gensler *et al.*, 1958; Hong *et al.*, 1979 and Rao *et al.*, 1962). The paucity of reports describing such conjugates of steroid molecules and antitumor agents from plant or fermentation sources prompted the preparation and biological evaluation of conjugates from suitable estrogen derivatives and selected vinca alkaloids described in this paper.

The discovery of vinblastine (VLB), an anti-proliferative factor in leaf extracts of the periwinkle plant *(Catharanthus roseus G. Don, Vinca Rosea Lin.)* at the University of Western Ontario (Cutts *et al.*, 1960) and, concurrently, at the Lilly Research Laboratories (Johnson *et al.*, 1959) was soon followed by the discovery in these extracts of vincristine (VCR) and additional dimeric indole-dihydro-indole alkaloids possessing striking activity against the murine P1534 leukemia (Svoboda, 1961). Thus, VLB given ip for nine successive days in a dose range of 0.1-0.5 mg/kg appreciably increased survival of treated mice over that of controls without producing long-term survivors. VCR at 0.1-0.25 mg/kg did produce long-term survivors (Johnson *et al.*, 1963). VCR also was shown to have activity against the Ridgway osteogenic sarcoma (ROS) and the Gardner lymphosar-coma (GLS), murine tumor systems that are insensitive to VLB (Barnett *et al.*, 1978; Johnson *et al.*, 1963). Additional murine tumor systems sensitive to both alkaloids include the P388 leukemia, the B16 melanoma, and others (Barnett et al., 1978; Johnson et al., 1963).

Mitotic arrest of mammalian cells in culture by Vinca alkaloids presents another facet of their biological activity. Mitotic accumulation of Chinese hamster cells by VCR (at 0.002 μg/ml) reveals a greater potency than that of VLB (active at 0.02 μg/ml) (Sweeney, et al., 1978). A similar potency for VCR and VLB is apparent in their affinity of binding to tubulin, an interaction deemed basic to their antimitotic effect (Sartorelli et al., 1969) and, presumably, to their antitumor acitivity.

This tubulin-based mechanism of Vinca alkaloid action has a significant, favorable therapeutic consequence, namely, the absence of an associated mutagenic-carcinogenic potential. While a number of clinically useful antitumor agents express their activity by interacting - covalently or non-covalently - with DNA function and carry a potential risk of carcinogenesis for the patient, the Vinca alkaloids, interacting non-covalently with tubulin, do not carry this risk. Lack of carcinogenic activity has been demonstrated for VLB in an animal model (Schmahl et al., 1970).

The molecular structures of VLB (I) and VCR (II) differ only in the nature of the substituent, a methyl group or a formyl group, respectively, on the vindoline N_a-atom (Neuss et al., 1964). Despite this "minor" structural difference, the two alkaloids differ substantially in clinical utility as well as in clinical toxicity (DeConti et al., 1975; Johnson et al., 1963). The chief use of VLB is in the treatment of patients with Hodgkin's disease, while VCR, often in combination, is widely used in the treatment of acute lymphocytic leukemia in childhood (DeVita et al., 1970). Bone marrow toxicity is a dose-limiting factor in clinical therapy with VLB, whereas VCR in children and in adults frequently produces a peripheral neuropathy which necessitates reduction of dosage or discontinuation of therapy (Grobe et al., 1972; Weiss et al., 1974).

A program of chemical modification of VLB at the Lilly Research Laboratories, initiated to prepare a VLB analog which - hopefully - would emulate the superior antitumor activity of VCR but lack its dose-limiting neurotoxicity, led to the selection of deacetyl vinblastine amide (vindesine) as a candidate for clinical evaluation (Barnett *et al.*, 1978),. Vindesine (VDS, III), one of more than forty analogs prepared (Conrad *et al.*, 1979), was found to possess optimum collective activity against several murine tumor systems used for its evaluation.

The experimental antitumor spectrum of VDS, including activity against the ROS and GLS systems, resembled that of VCR rather than that of VLB, the parent alkaloid used in its preparation. Against the B16 melanoma, a murine tumor system reported to be predictive for clinical activity (Venditti *et al.*, 1975), VDS was found to be more effective then VCR.

Vindesine was further evaluated in several experimental models designed for the estimation of its potential neurotoxicity relative to that of VCR. Results obtained in these models, involving inhibition of axoplasmic transport *in vitro* in the cat sciatic nerve (Iqbal *et al.*, 1979), cytological changes in new born rat brain cells in culture (King *et al.*, 1979), behavioral and neurological effects in the chicken and monkey (Todd *et al.*, 1979), uniformly point to a lower potential for neurotoxicity for VDS.

These observations together with toxicological (Todd *et al.*, 1976), metabolic (Culp *et al.*, 1977), and pharmacokinetic studies (Nelson *et al.*, 1979) encouraged the clinical evaluation of VDS at the Lilly Laboratories for Clinical Research (Dyke *et al.*, 1977) and at various cancer centers in the USA and abroad (Dyke *et al.*, 1979). Phase I and II clinical trial reports indicate VDS to be an active oncolytic agent (Dyke *et al.*, 1977) producing a high proportion of remissions in patients with acute lymphocytic leukemia (Dyke *et al.*, 1979). Clinically, VDS appears to be less neurotoxic than VCR and, generally, its administration has not had to be discontinued because of neurotoxicity (Dyke *et al.*, 1977). The limiting side effect of VDS in therapeutic dose regimen is neutropenia (Dyke *et al.*, 1979).

In some advanced acute lymphocytic leukemia patients resistant to VCR, VDS has induced remissions and, thus, appears to lack cross-resistance with VCR (Dyke *et al.*, 1979; Gralla *et al.*, 1979; Krivit *et al.*, 1978; Mathe *et al.*, 1978). Results obtained with VDS in patients with small cell and non-small cell carcinoma of the lung have encouraged further studies of VDS in combination with cis-dichlorodiamineplatinum (II) in this disease (Dyck *et al.*, 1977; Gralla *et al.*, 1979).

The preliminary clinical results with VDS obtained thus far include a number of potential benefits not anticipated from the experimental findings. These benefits, which include the possible activity of VDS in lung cancer and the lack of cross resistance between VDS and VCR mentioned above, encourage further research efforts to enhance or expand the therapeutic efficacy of the oncolytic vinca alkaloids through chemical modification. With regard to the present work in particular, phase II study of vindesine in breast carcinoma (Smith *et al.*, 1978 & 1979) prompted the synthesis and biological evaluation of estrogen-vinca alkaloid conjugates.

Rather than view the proposed estrogen-vinca conjugates as examples of "double-drug" agents, we tend to look on the estrogen moiety as a carrier for the oncolytic alkaloid moiety which hopefully would affect distribution of the latter to estrogen-receptive cell types. Naturally, the role of the estrogen moiety itself on tumor growth requires separate investigation ranging between agonist and antagonist estrogen structures. When seen in this way as a carrier-type approach, the vinca-estrogen conjugate effort parallels similar other projects linking antitumor agents to macromolecules, e.g. adriamycin-DNA complexes (Trouet *et al.*, 1979) and adriamycin-tumor cell antibody conjugates (Levy *et al.*, 1975).

At this early stage of the project, it cannot be ascertained whether a biodegradable connecting chain linking the two molecules is to be preferred, or a non-biodegradable chain. In the latter case, the conjugate would hopefully express the derived biological function(s) of the intact molecules, whereas in the former, gradual release of both moieties resulting from enzymic or chemical hydrolysis would be the preferred mode of action.

The specific aim of this research is to attach an estrogen covalently through an intervening chain to the "lower" (vindoline) moiety of a dimeric vinca alkaloid. As described above, certain structural changes involving the hydroxyl and carboxylic functions in the vindoline moiety of VLB (or VDS) can be made without the loss of experimental antitumor activity, wheras the consequences of such changes in the velbanamine ("upper") moiety appear to be less predictable (Conrad *et al.*, 1979; Gerzon *et al.*, 1979). Thus deacetyl vinblastine acid hydrazide (IV) (Barnett *et al.*, 1978), a versatile, readily available vindoline-modified derivative became the logical choice for the vinca portion of the conjugates in our initial experiments.

In the preparation of affinity columns for the purification of estrogen receptor, those in which the attachment between agarose and the steroid was through the A ring were ineffective either because they exhibited poor affinity for the receptor or because they were unstable in the presence of cytoplasmic protein (Sica *et al.,* 1973). On the other hand, columns in which the attachment was through positions 6 or 17 were highly effective for purification of estrogen receptor from calf uterus. Assuming estrogen receptor in breast to have similar affinity, we elected to employ estrone carboxymethoxylamine (V) (Erlanger *et al.,* 1959), estradiol 3-benzoate 17-hemisuccinate (VI) and 6-ketoestradiol 6-carboxymethoxylamine (VII) (Dean *et al.,* 1971) as the steroid moiety.

I   R=CH₃   VLB

II R=CHO VCR

III R=H   VDS

IV R=NH₂

Results and Discussion

The carboxymethoxylamine derivative V of estrone was converted to its methyl ester VIII, which reacted with anhydrous hydrazine to give the acid hydrazide IX in good yield. Deacetylvinblastine hydrazide (IV) was converted to the corresponding azide X with nitrous acid. The azide, without purification, was treated with the acid hydrazide IX in dimethysulfoxide. The product XI was purified by column chromatography and by preparative thin layer chromatography. Estrone carboxymethoxylamine deacetylvinblastine acid hydrazide conjugate (XI) exhibited an ultraviolet maximum at 270 nm, characteristic of vinca alkaloids. It binds to estrogen receptor about one sixtieth as strong as estradiol (Fig. 1).

As a prelude to coupling in the opposite direction, that is, activated steroid to vinca alkaloid, a model reaction was carried out on benzyl amine and the acid azide from estradiol 3-benzoate 17-hemisuccinate (XII). The latter was converted to the acid chloride with thionyl chloride. After removal of excess SOCl₂, the crude acid chloride reacted smoothly with sodium azide in dimethylsulfoxide to give the acid azide XIV. Without purification it was treated with a tetrahydrofuran solution of benzyl amine. The product, estradiol 3-benzoate 17-hemisuccinate N-benzylamide (XV), exhibited ir and nmr spectra consistent with the expected structure. All attempts to hydrolyze XV selectively at the 3-position with potassium carbonate failed; estradiol was inevitably obtained.

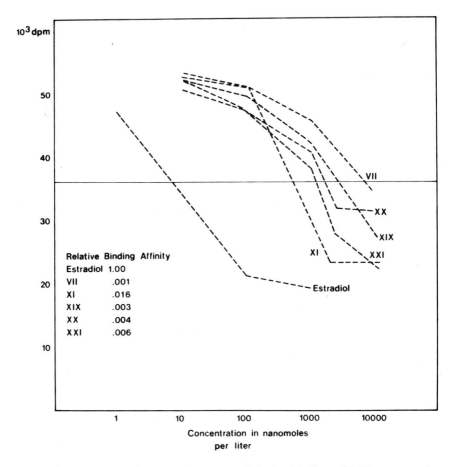

Fig. 1: Binding to Estrogen Receptor. Relative binding affinities were calculated from the concentrations at which 50% of the receptor is bound. VII, 6-Ketoestradiol 6-carboxymethoxylamine; XI, estrone carboxymethoxylamine deacetylvinblastine acid hydrazide conjugate; XIX, 6-ketoestradiol 6-carboxymethoxylamine 17-acetate; XX, 6-ketoestradiol 6-carboxymethoxylamine 17-acetate deacetylvinblastine acid hydrazide conjugate; XXI, 6-ketoestradiol 6-carboxymethoxylamine deacetylvinblastine acid hydrazide conjugate.

The same acid azide XIV reacted similarly with deacetylvinblastine acid hydrazide (IV) to give estradiol 3-benzoate 17-hemisuccinate deacetylvinblastine acid hydrazide conjugate (XVII). It exhibited ir and uv spectra consistent with the structure, and further support comes from its alkaline hydrolysis to estradiol.

The mitotic accumulation assay is illustrated in Fig. 2. The G_1/G_0 peak (Horan et al., 1977), major peak in the control, is largely

XI

replaced by a G_2 + M peak by vinblastine (I). Making allowance for molecular weight, XVII exhibited anti-mitotic activity of the order of vinblastine. It was assumed that XVII probably would not bind to estrogen receptor because both hydroxyls at C-3 and at C-17 are protected in the form of ester linkages. It was examined for *in vivo* estrogenic activity, however, and was found to possess only minimal activity (Table I).

In order to synthesize a conjugate with both hydroxyl groups of estradiol free, 6-ketoestradiol diacetate (XVIII) was converted to the carboxymethoxylamine derivative XIX (losing the 3-acetate group in

TABLE I
Estrogen Assay of Estradiol 3-Benzoate 17-Hemisuccinate Deacetylvinblastine
Acid Hydrazide Conjugate (XVIII)

	Dose	Av. Uterine Wt.
Control		10.6 mg
XVII	300 µg/day	25.6 (8 out of 10 dead)
	100 µg/day	35.8 (2 out of 10 dead)
Estradiol	1 µg/day	50.3

Compounds were administered for 3 days by s.c. injection of the sample in corn
oil, using immature mice.

the process) and condensed with deacetylvinblastive acid hydrazide
(IV) in the presence of dicyclohexylcarbodiimide. The product XX
was hydrolysed with alcoholic KOH at room temperature to 6-keto-
estradiol 6-carboxymethoxylamine deacetylvinblastine acid hydrazide conjugate (XXI). Both XX and XXI underwent acid hydrolysis to
6-ketoestradiol (XXII), identical with that from 6-ketoestradiol diacetate (XVIII).

6-Ketoestradiol 6-carboxymethoxylamine (VII) binds to estrogen
receptor one-thousandth as strong as estradiol (Fig. 1). This may be
compared with the report that the dissociation constant of receptor-
bound VII is fifty thousand times as large as that of estradiol
(Schmahl et al., 1970). Binding of estradiol is 300 times as strong as
that of the 17-acetate XIX, 160 times as strong as that of the conjugate XXI, and 250 times that of its 17-acetate (XX) (Fig. 1).

As would be expected, neither 6-ketoestradiol 6-carboxymethoxy-lamine (VII) nor its 17-acetate (XIX) inhibit mitosis (Fig. 2), but both XX and XXI are active. Thus, in the three conjugates examined, the anti-mitotic activity of the vinca alkaloid remains unimpaired with the steroid attached.

Conclusions and Extension of Research

Though our initial exploratory results reported here encourage

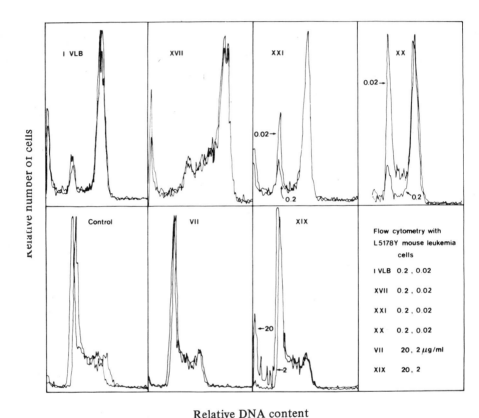

Relative DNA content

Fig. 2: In Vitro Kinetics of L5178Y Mouse Leukemia Cells I, Vinblastine, (conc. in g/ml); VII, 6-ketoestradiol carboxymethoxylamine; XVII, estradiol 3-benzo-ate 17-hemisuccinate deacetylvinblastine acid hydrazide conjugate, XX, 6-keto-estradiol 6-carboxymethoxylamine 17-acetate deacetylvinblastine acid hydrazide conjugate; XXI, 6-ketoestradiol 6-carboxymethoxylamine deacetylvinblastine acid hydrazide conjugate.

further pursuit of the vinca-estrogen conjugates, definition and expansion of the chemical work is planned. Specifically, the structures of the vinca and estrogen moieties need to be varied, as well as the type of chemical linkage of the connecting chain, in order to vary the degree and susceptibility to biodegradation, and hopefully, to enhance the binding to estrogen receptor.

Material and methods

Melting points were taken on a Thomas Hoover melting point apparatus and are corrected. Infrared spectra were recorded in mineral oil mulls on a Perkin-Elmer 247 Spectrophotometer. Ultraviolet spectra were recorded in MeOH solution on a Cary 15 Spectrophotometer. NMR spectra were recorded in CDCL$_3$ solution on a Varian Associates T-60 or HA-100 instrument. Chemical shifts are recorded in parts per million (δ) relative to $(CH_3)_4$ Si as internal standard. Microanalyses were obtained from Galbraith Laboratories, Knoxville, Tennessee.

Estrone Carboxymethoxylamine Deacetylvinblastine Acid Hydrazide Conjugate (XI)

A solution of 6.698 g of estrone carboxymethoxylamine (V) in 5 ml of conc HCl and 200 ml of methanol was stirred at reflux for 2 hr, decanted from a trace of insoluble solid, and refrigerated overnight. Filtering gave the crude *methyl ester VIII,* 5.763 g, m.p. 179-184°C. The analytical sample, recrystallized in methanol, m.p. 183-184, ir 3350 (OH), 1740 (C=O), 1620, 1516, 1250, 1100, 1075, 1035, 920, 886, 825, 675 cm^{-1}, calcd for $C_{20}H_{27}NO_4$: C, 69.54; H, 7.88; N, 4.06. Found: C, 70.05; H, 7.79; N. 3.89. A mixture of 5.055 g of estrone carbomethoxymethoxylamine and 30 ml of hydrazine (97%) was stirred at room temperature overnight. The solution was diluted with 50 ml of H_2O, precipitating the crude product. 4.718 g, m.p. 264-266°. Recrystallization in methanol-dimethylformamide (3:1) gave *estrone carboxymethoxylamine hydrazide (IX),* m.p. 265-266° (d), ir 3370 (OH), 3280 and 3180 (NH), 1675 (C=O), 1615, 1505, 1239, 1110, 1075, 1050, 930, 918, 820 cm^{-1}, calcd for $C_{19}H_{27}N_3O_4$: C, 67.20: H, 7.61: N, 11.75. Found: C, 67.26; H, 7.63; N, 11.65. Deacetylvinblastine hydrazide (Conrad *et al.,* 1979) (IV, 460 mg, 0.60 mM) was dissolved in 25 ml of 1 N HCl and the solution then cooled to 4°. Dry $NaNO_2$ (45 mg, 0.65 mM) was added with stirring. After 5 min, 5% aqueous $NaHCO_3$ was added until the pH was approximately 8. The resulting suspension was extracted with 3 x 40 ml of CH_2Cl_2. The extracts were combined, dried over anhydrous Na_2SO_4, and filtered, then concentrated to 65 ml. To this solution was added a solution of 108 mg (0.30 mM) of estrone carboxymethoxylamine hydrazide (IX) in 23 ml of dimethylsulfoxide (DMSO). After standing at room temperature overnight, the solution was diluted with 65 ml of CH_2Cl_2, washed twice with 5% aqueous $NaHCO_3$, dried over Na_2SO_4, filtered and evaporated, leaving 435 mg of residue. It was taken up in CH_2Cl_2 (40 mg of starting acid hydrazide did not dissolve) and chromatographed on 13 g of Al_2O_3. After preliminary fractions eluted by CH_2Cl_2 and by up to 4% MeOH in CH_2Cl_2, 52 mg of crude product (A) was eluted by 8-12% MeOH in CH_2Cl_2, and another portion (B), 24 mg, was eluted by 16-20% MeOH in CH_2Cl_2. Portion A was dissolved in $HCCl_3$ and separated by preparative TLC (silica gel) in 5% MeOH in CH_2Cl_2. A band with R_f 0.4-0.5 was combined with a similar band from the preparative TLC of B, to give the *product (XI),* 4.5 mg, uv$_{max}$ 270 nm.

Estradiol 3-Benzoate 17-Hemisuccinate N-Benzylamide (XV).

A solution of 6.12 g of estradiol 3-benzoate 17-hemisuccinate (XII) in 20 ml of $SOCl_2$ was stirred at approximately 40° for 2 hr, then evaporated with suction to remove excess $SOCl_2$. One g of the crude acid chloride was added to a stirred solution of 1 g of NaN_3 in 25 ml of DMSO. After 80 min at room temperature, 1 g of benzyl amine in 5 ml of tetrahydrofuran (THF) was added. After 1 hr, H_2O was added to turbidity and the mixture was refrigerated 3 hr. The crude product, 855 mg, m.p. 76-97° could not be crystallized from acetone-H_2O, so it was dissolved in petroleum ether and chromatographed on 26 g of Al_2O_3. The portion, 214 mg, eluted by CH_2Cl_2-ether (4:1), was recrystallized from acetone-H_2O to give the *N-benzyl amide XV*, m.p. 149-151, ir 3330 (NH), 1730 (ester C=O), 1646 (amide C-O), 1540, 1274, 1235, 1180, 1066, 720 cm^{-1}, 1H NMR δ 0.84 (3H, s, 18-CH_3), 2.6 (4H, q, succinate CH_2's), 4.42 (2H, d, benzyl CH_2), 6.8-8.3 (13H, m, aromatic), calcd for $C_{36}H_{38}NO_5$:C, 76.57; H, 6.78; N, 2.48. Found: C, 76.28; H, 6.99; N, 2.38. Hydrolysis of the N-benzylamide with K_2CO_3 in aqueous MeOH gave estradiol, identified by m.p. ir and TLC.

Estradiol 3-Benzoate 17-Hemisuccinate

Deacetylvinblastine Acid Hydrazide Conjugate (XVII).

A solution of 80 mg (0.1 mM) of deacetylvinblastine acid hydrazide (IV) in 3 ml of DMSO was added dropwise to a stirred solution of estradiol 3-benzoate 17-hemisuccinate acid azide (XIV), prepared from 100 mg, 0.2 mM, of the acid chloride (see above), in 10 ml of DMSO and 25 ml of THF. The solution was stirred 64 hr at room temperature, concentrated on the Rotovap to 30 ml, diluted with 50 ml of CH_2Cl_2 and washed with aqueous 5% $NaHCO_3$. The organic layer was evaportaed on the Rotovap, the residual oil was dissolved in acetone and resulting solution was made turbid with H_2 and refrigated. Filtering gave an A crop, 66 mg, ir 3460 (OH), 1735 (ester C=O), 1620 (amide C=O), 1500, 1276, 1258, 1220, 1180, 1158, 1070, 720 cm^{-1}, uv$_{max}$ 270 nm, and from the filtrate, a B crop, 15 mg. A 45 mg mixture of A and B was purified by preparative TLC on silica in 14% MeOH in CH_2Cl_2. The product, conjugate XVII, 14 mg, was recovered from a band R_f 0.25 to 0.63. Hydrolysis of a portion of the conjugate in methanolic KOH at room temperature overnight, dilution with H_2O and extraction with CH_2Cl_2 gave estradiol, identified by uv and TLC.

6-Ketoestradiol 6-Carboxymethoxylamine Deacetylvinblastine Acid Hydrazide Conjugate (XXI).

6-Ketoestradiol diacetate (XVIII) (Dean *et al.*, 1971) was treated with carboxymethoxylamine hemihydrochloride, forming the expected derivative except that the 3-acetate group was cleaved in the process. A solution of 222 mg. (0.55 mM) of 6-ketoestradiol 17-acetate carboxymethoxylamine (XIX) 383 mg, (0.50 mM) of deacetylvinblastine hydrazide (IV) and 113 mg (0.55 mM) of dicyclohexylcarbodiimide in 15 ml of CH_2Cl_2 stood at room temperature overnight. A small amount of dicyclohexylurea (DCU) was filtered out, the CH_2Cl_2 was evaporated, the residue was taken up in acetone and more DCU removed by filtration. The filtrate was made turbid with H_2O and refrigerated, depositing 378 mg of an amorphous solid, m.p. 191-201°, ir 3400-3200 (OH unresolved from NH), 1720 (ester C=O), 1652 and 1620 (amide C=O), 1260, 1085, 1050, 1020, 880, 750 cm^{-1}, and a second crop, 51 mg, m.p. 196-201°. A portion of the first crop was dissolved in benzene and reprecipitated by the addition of petroleum ether, giving *conjugate XX*, m.p. 216-223°, 1H NMR δ 2.05 (3H, s, acetate CH_3), 2.62 (1H, s, C21H), 2.81 (3H, s, CH_3N), 3.60 (3H, s, CO_2CH_3), 3.76 (3H, s, CH_3O), 4.14 (1H, s, C17H), 5.76 (2H, m, olefinic H), 6.05 (1H, s, C12H), 6.58 (1H, s, C9H), 6.80 (1H, s, aromatic H), 7.13 (3H, m, C9'H, C10'H, C11'H), 7.50 (1H, s, C12'H), 8.05 (1H, s, NH) (numbers refer to the alkaloid moiety), uv$_{max}$ 264nm.

A solution of 198 mg of the conjugate XX in 30 ml of EtOH and 30 ml of 2N KOH stood at room temperature overnight. The solution was diluted with 200 ml of H_2O and extracted thrice with CH_2Cl_2. Drying and evaproating left 99 mg of residue which was purified by preparative TLC on silica in 7% MeOH in CH_2Cl_2. The portion with R_f 0.25 to 0.50 was recovered, *conjugate XXI*, 22.5 mg, m.p. 143-153°, uv$_{max}$ 264 nm.

When examined by paper electrophoresis, VII and p-nitrophenylacetic acid (for reference) both migrated toward the anode, while XXI remained at the origin, in keeping with the assigned structure.

Acknowledgments

We are most grateful to Drs. Russel Kraay and Larry Black, Lilly Research Laboratories, for the receptor binding measurements and for the estrogen assay. We are also indebted to Mr. George Boder, Lilly Research Laboratories, for the mitotic accumulation measurements. We sincerely appreciate the gift of deacetyl vinblastine hydrazide from Lilly Research Laboratories.

References

Barnett, C. J., Cullinan, G. J., Gerzon, K., Hoying, R. C., Jones, W. E., Newlon, W. M., Poore, G. A., Robinson, R. L., Sweeney, M. J., Todd, R. C., Dyke, R. W., and Nelson, R. L. (1978). *J. Med. Chem.* **21**, 88.

Carroll, R. I., Philip, A., Blackwell, J. T., Taylor, D. J., and Wall, M. E. (1972). *J. Med. Chem.* **15**, 1158.

Conrad, R. A., Cullinan, G. J., Gerzon, K., and Poore, G. A. (1979). *J. Med. Chem.* **22**, 391.

Culp, H. W., Daniels, W. D., and McMahon, R. E. (1977). *Cancer Res.* **37**, 3053.

Cutts, J. H., Beer, C. T., and Noble, R. L. (1960). *Cancer Res.* **20**, 1023.

Dean, P. D. G., Exley, D., and Johnson, M. W. (1971). *Steroids* **18**, 593.

DeConti, R. C., and Creasey, W. C., "*The Catharanthus Alkaloids,*" W. I. Taylor and N. R. Farnsworth, Editors, Marcel Decker, New York, N. Y., 1975, p. 237-278.

DeVita, V. T. Jr., Serpick, A. A., and Carbone, P. P. (1970). *Ann. Intern. Med.* **73**, 881.

Dyke, R. W., and Nelson, R. L. (1977). *Cancer Treatm. Rev.* **4**, 135.

Dyke, R. W., Nelson, R. L., and Brade, W. P. (1979). *Cancer Chemother. Pharmacol.* **2**, 229, and further reports in this issue.

Erlanger, B. F., Borek, F., Beiser, S. M., and Lieberman, S. (1959). *J. Biol. Chem.* **234**, 1090.

Gensler, W. J., and Sherman, G. M. (1958). *J. Org. Chem.* **23**, 1227.

Gerzon, K., Dimeric Catharanthus Alkaloids, *in* "*Development of Anticancer Drugs Based on Natural Product Prototypes,*" J. M. Cassidy and J. C. Douros, Editors, Academic Press, in press.

Gralla, R. J., Tan, C. T. C. (1979). *Cancer Chemother. Pharmacol,* **2**, 247.

Grobe, H., and Palm, D. (1972). *Monatsschr. Kinderheilkd.* **120**, 23.

Horan, P. K., and Wheeless, L. L., Jr. (1977). *Science* **198**, 149.

Hong, C. I., Nechaev, A., and West, C. R. (1979). 178th ACS National Meeting, Washington, D. C., Sept. 10-13, MEDI 43.

Iqbal, Z., and Ochs, S. (1979). *J. Neurochem.* **33**: in press.

Johnson, I. S., Armstrong, J. G., Gorman, M., and Burnett, J. P. (1963). *Cancer Res.* **23**, 1390.

Johnson, I. S., Hargrove, W. W., Harris, P. N., Wright, H. F. and Boder, G. B. (1966). *Cancer Res.* **26**, 2431.

Johnson, I. S., Wright, H. F., and Svoboda, G. H. (1959). *J. Lab. Clin. Med.* **54**, 830.

King, K., and Boder, G. B. (1979). *Cancer Chemother. Pharmacol,* **2**, 239.

Korenman, S. G., Perrin, L. E., and McCallum, T. P. (1969). *J. Clin. Endocrin. Metab.* **29**, 879.

Krivit, W., Hammond, D. (1978). *Curr. Chemother.* **2**, 1331.

Levy, R., Hurwitz, E., Maron, R., Arnon, R., and Sela, M. (1975). *Cancer Res.* **35**, 1182-1186.

Mathe, G., Misset, J. L., De Vassal, F., Hayat, M., Machover, D., Bel Poome, D., Schwarzenberg, L., Ribaud, P., Musset, M., and Jasmin, C. (1978). *Cancer Treatm. Rep.* **62**, 805.

Nelson, R. L., Dyke, R. W., and Root, M. A. (1979). *Cancer Chemother. Pharmacol.* **2**, 243.

Neuss, N., Gorman, M., Hargrove, W. W., Cone, N. J., Biemann, K., Buchl, G., and Manning, R. (1964). *J. Amer. Chem. Soc.* **86**, 1440.

Rao, G. V., and Price, C. C. (1962). *J. Org. Chem.* **27**, 205.

Sartorelli, A. C., and Creasey, W. A. (1969). *Ann. Rev. Pharmacol.* **9**, 51.
Schmahl, D., and Osswald, H., (1970). *Arzneim. Forsch.* **20**, 1461.
Sica, V., Parikh, I., Nola, E., Puca, G. A., and Cuatrecassas, P. (1973). *J. Biol. Chem.* **248**, 6543.
Smith, I. E., Hedley, D. W., Powless, T. J., and McElwain, T. J. (1978). *Cancer Treatm. Rep.* **62**, 1427.
Smith, I. E., and Powles, T. J. (1979). *Cancer Chemother. Pharmacol.* **2**, 261.
Svoboda, G. H. (1961). Lloydia **24**, 173.
Sweeney, M. J., Boder, G. B., Cullinan, G. J., Culp, H. W., Daniels, W. D., Dyke, R. W., Gerzon, K., McMahon, R. E., Nelson, R. L., Poore, G. A., and Todd, G. C. (1978). *Cancer. Res.* **38**, 2886.
Todd, G. C., Gibson, W. R., and Morton, D. M. (1976). *J. Toxicol. Environ, Health,* **1**, 843.
Todd, G. C., Griffing, W. J., Gibson, W. R., and Morton, D. M. (1979). *Cancer Treatm. Rep.* **63**, 35.
Trouet, A., and Sokal, G. (1979). *Cancer Treatm. Rep.* **63**, 895.
Venditti, J. M. in *"Pharmacological Basis of Cancer Chemotherapy"* Williams and Wilkins Company, Baltimore, MD. 1975, p. 245-270.
Weiss, H. D., Walker, M. D., and Wiernik P. H. (1974). *New Engl. J. Med.* **291**, 127.

Discussion

Wittliff: What are the cells that you used to study the mitotic inhibition?

Blickenstaff: L 5178 Y mouse leukemia cells.

Wittliff: Do they have estrogen receptors?

Blickenstaff: Not necessarily. I showed them because of the background of the Vinca alkaloids on those cells.

Wittliff: What is the evidence that the molecule is intact when it elicits its antimitotic effect?

Blickenstaff: We only know that it is intact when it is dissolved in the medium. I suppose there is a possibility that it could undergo splitting, although the linkage is a fairly stable one. It takes strong acid to cleave it.

Wittliff: Have you extracted the compound from the cell?

Blickenstaff: No, we have not. So we don't have any direct evidence that it is still intact.

Morgan: Why did you take vinca alkaloids? As far as I know they are not very effective against hormone dependent tumors.

Blickenstaff: They are not normally used in that way. That's very true. They are used in leukemia. However there are some very recent studies with Vincristine-Vindesine on breast carcinomas which show that they do have some effect, perhaps not as good as some other compounds. The advantage is that they don't have some of the harmful effects of the other compounds. We didn't choose them because they are especially good for hormone dependent tumors, but for other reasons.

Borgna: Did you try to use a longer spacer.

Blickenstaff: No, we haven't tried any other connectors but we thought about this. An ethylene diamine spacer for instance would be a good one.

Könyves: What is the solubility of these compounds?

Blickenstaff: They are not water soluble. They are soluble in alcohol, in acetone, DMSO, not in THF. There is one thing I forgot to mention: the second compound that we made was shown to have very weak estrogenic activity and was dissolved in oil to administer it. I don't know how soluble it was but it was soluble enough that it could be administered in corn oil.

N-MUSTARD GROUPS LINKED TO ESTROGENS: PROBLEMS OF SYNTHESIS AND RECEPTOR AFFINITY

H. HAMACHER, B. BORMANN, E. CHRIST

Institute for Drugs
Federal Health Office
Berlin, W. Germany

Introduction

The rational design of new drugs with high selective activity is an old aim of the medicinal chemist. With regard to antineoplastic agents, selective activity means a cytotoxic effect of drugs on the tumor cells without or with only a limited influence on normal tissues. At the present stage we are far from the aim of highly selective antitumor drugs, particularly from their development by rational concepts. Most of the chemotherapeutic agents available for cancer treatment have been found by chance or by large screening programmes, and cytotoxic selectivity for tumor cells of most of these drugs is rather low.

Two basic principles are available to the medicinal chemist working in the field of developing new antitumor drugs by a rational design:
- selection by differences in metabolism of tumor and normal cells
- selection by a particular pharmacokinetic property of cytotoxic agents (accumulation in malignant cells).

Both principles which cannot be clearly distinguished, have engaged a lot of chemists all over the world. In some cases, work has resulted in drugs useful for treatment of human cancers.

Work based on the pharmacokinetic principle of selection frequently uses physiological carriers which are linked to different cytotoxic groups. Among the physiological carriers, estrogen hormones seem to have a good chance of increasing the tumor cell selectivity of cytotoxic groups for the following reasons:

1. A high proportion of human cancers contain estrogen receptors.

2. Estrogen hormone molecules as well as some synthetic estrogens such as diethylstilbestrol or hexestrol show a high binding affinity to estrogen receptors.
3. The transport mechanism of the carrier-receptor complexes could result in the accumulation of cytotoxic estrogen derivatives in the nucleus of target cells which is the potential site of action, particularly for alkylating groups.

Synthesis of cytotoxic estrogens

Most of the cytotoxic estrogen derivatives described in the literature have been prepared by esterification of the hydroxyl groups of the estrogen carrier with suitable derivatives of alkylating carboxylic acids. Examples of such compounds are ICI 85 966, estradiol mustard, and estramustine.

The synthesis of compounds of this type is relatively easy. The available estrogen carriers can be transformed into the corresponding mustard derivatives by simple reactions (Carrol *et al.*, 1972, Larionov *et al.*, 1968). The disadvantage of these compounds is the instability of their ester groups under physiological conditions. It is possible that the alkylating groups is split off before the drug reaches the tumor cell.

Therefore, our aim was to attach the cytotoxic groups to the estrogen carrier by a stable linkage whose cleavage under physiological

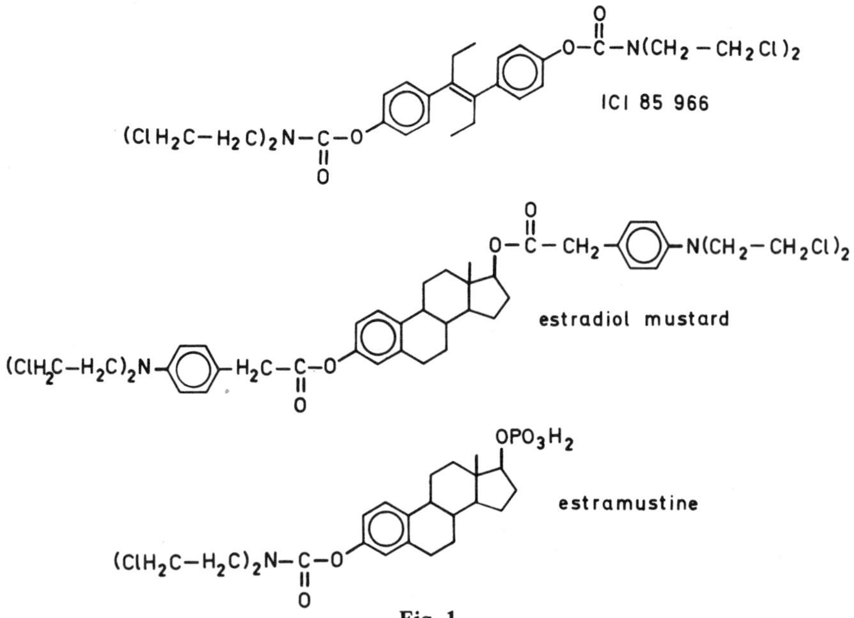

Fig. 1

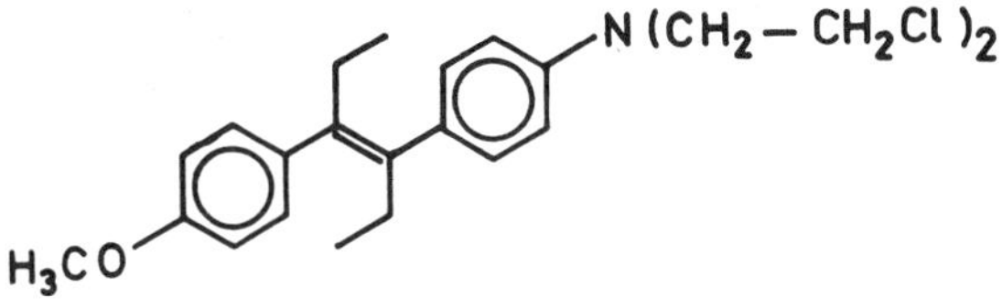

Fig. 2

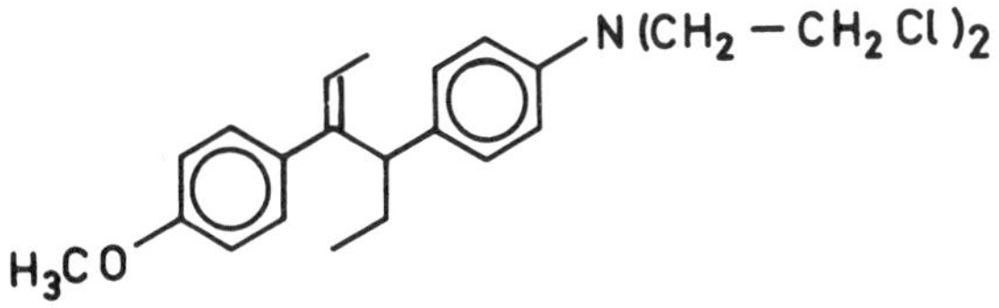

conditions was unlikely. Our first compounds of this type, 1 and 2, prepared by total synthesis (Hamacher *et al.*, 1977), are derivatives of diethylstilbestrol or its isomeric 2-hexene compound. Both alkylating derivatives contain an N-mustard function instead of one hydroxyl group. The second hydroxyl group of the carrier is protected, being a methyl ether. 1 and 2, as well as the compounds of the ester type, do not contain free hydroxyl groups which are important for the binding process at the estrogen receptor site. They have been proved to lack affinity for the estrogen receptor.

With regard to the required receptor affinity our next aim was to synthesize cytotoxic compounds with free hydroxyl groups. Our first compounds of this type were 3, 4, 5, and 6 (Fig. 3 & 4) which were prepared from diethylstilbestrol, hexestrol, and estrone, respectively (Hamacher, 1978 & 1979). These N-mustard derivatives, particularly 5 and 6, can bind to the estrogen receptor as will be shown in another report to be presented later during this Workshop.

In a further series of experiments we tried to prepare the diethylstilbestrol derivative 7 (Fig. 5) with an N-mustard group in ortho position of one hydroxyl group by total synthesis. This synthesis proved to be extremely difficult and the desired compound 7 could not yet be obtained (Fig. 6). Starting material for the conceived synthesis was 2-phenylbutyric acid which was first converted into ethyl 2-(4-hydroxyphenyl)butyrate by esterification with ethanol, nitration in 4-position of the phenyl ring, reduction of the nitro to the amino group, diazotation, and transformation of the diazonium into the phenolic hydroxyl group. In a second nitration step a nitro

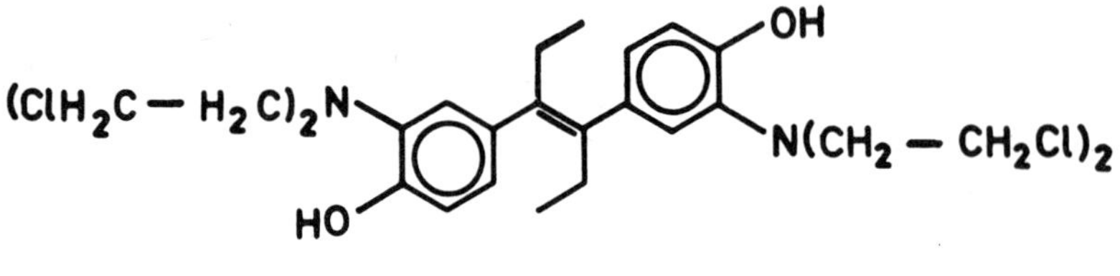

3

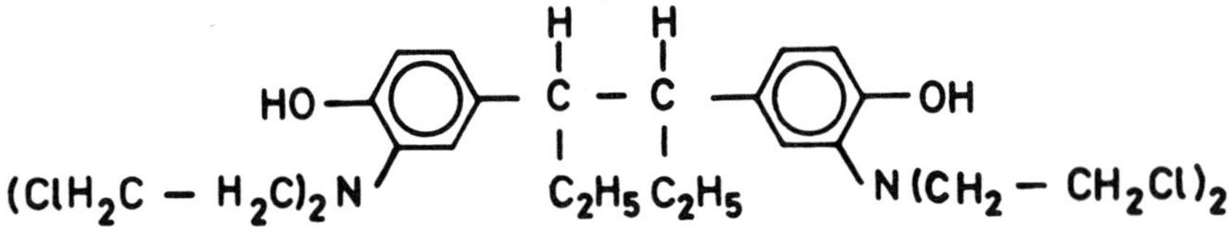

4

Fig. 3

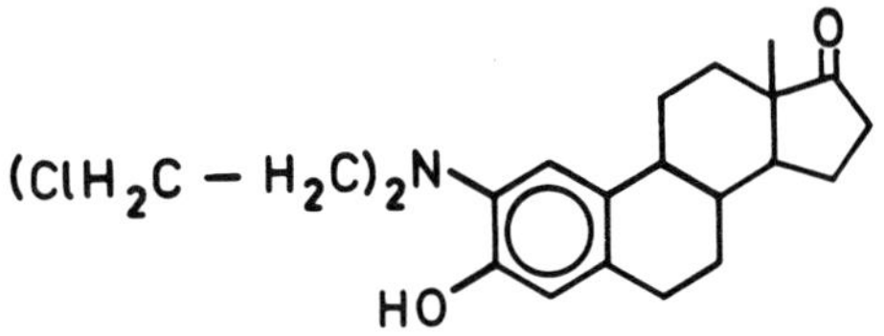

5

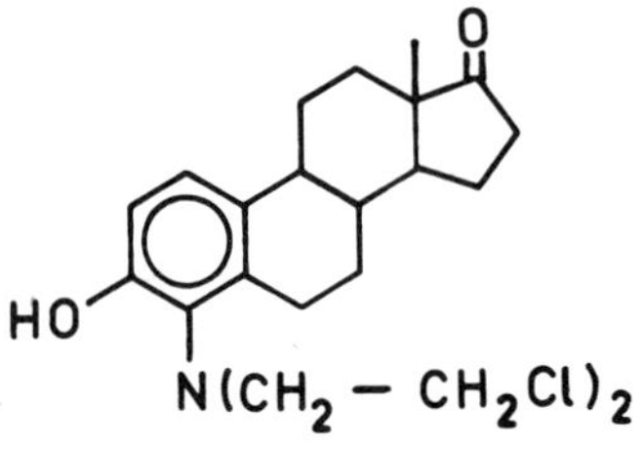

6

Fig. 4

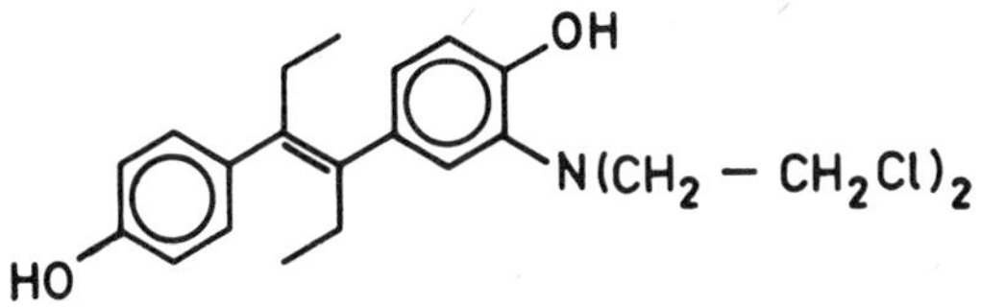

7

Fig. 5

group was introduced in the ortho position of the phenolic hydroxyl group. The latter was then protected for the further course of synthesis by methylation.

The second phenyl ring was introduced in a Friedel Crafts reaction with anisol. The resulting ketone was converted, by means of magnesium ethyl bromide, into the tertiary alcohol, 8.

The next step proved to be critical. Instead of the expected stilbene derivative 9, the isomeric 2-hexene compound 10 was obtained. Nevertheless, 2-hexene derivatives, being analogous to diethylstilbestrol with additional substituents in the phenyl rings, have antiestrogenic properties as has been demonstrated by Clark and O'Donnel (Clark *et al.*, 1965) and thus seem to be bound to estrogen receptors. Therefore, we converted the 2-hexene compound, 10 to the corresponding N-mustard derivative, 11 by reaction with ethylene oxide and chlorination of the resulting hydroxyethylamino intermediate. The corresponding demethylated N-mustard derivative could not be obtained due to the very low overall yield and to difficulties at some critical steps of the total synthesis.

The most promising cytotoxic estrogen derivative synthesized in our laboratory seems to be the estradiol derivative 12 with an N-mustard group in the 6-position of the steroid system. After various fruitless trials we obtained 12 in very small amounts by the route shown in Fig. 7.

Estradiol was acetylated and 3,17-diacetylestradiol converted into the 6-keto derivative by oxidation with chromium (VI) oxide. The ketone was transformed into the oxime whose selective reduction to the corresponding amine is difficult. A diacetylated 6-aminoestradiol whose stereochemistry is not yet clear was prepared by mild reduction of the oxime with zinc and ammonia in ethanol. Conversion of the 6-aminoderivative into the corresponding N-mustard compound was carried out by hydroxyethylation, deacetylation and subsequent chlorination of the resulting hydroxyethylamino product. Due to the very low amount of 12 (overall yield 1 - 2 %), biological testing of this compound could not yet be carried out.

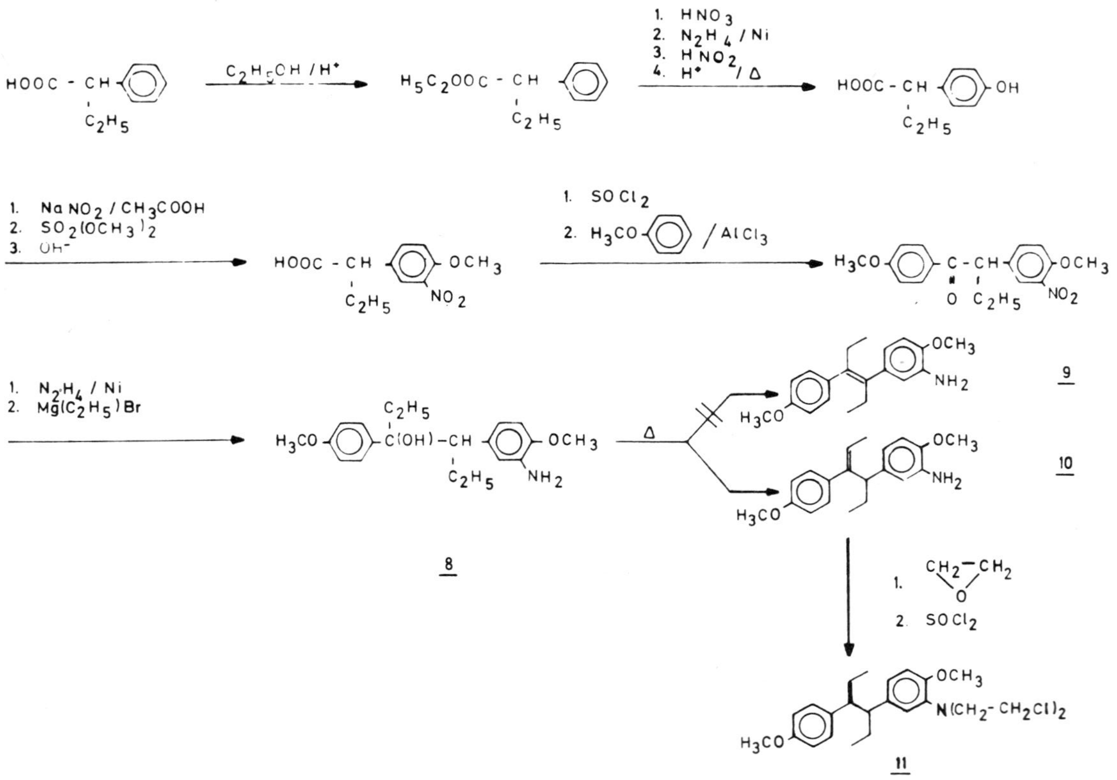

HOOC-CH(C$_2$H$_5$)C$_6$H$_5$

$\xrightarrow{\text{C}_2\text{H}_5\text{OH} / \text{H}^+}$

H$_5$C$_2$OOC-CH(C$_2$H$_5$)C$_6$H$_5$

1. HNO$_3$
2. N$_2$H$_4$/Ni
3. HNO$_2$
4. H$^+$/Δ

$\rightarrow$ HOOC-CH(C$_2$H$_5$)-C$_6$H$_4$-OH

1. NaNO$_2$/CH$_3$COOH
2. SO$_2$(OCH$_3$)$_2$
3. OH$^-$

HOOC-CH(C$_2$H$_5$)-C$_6$H$_3$(OCH$_3$)(NO$_2$)

1. SOCl$_2$
2. H$_3$CO-C$_6$H$_5$ / AlCl$_3$

H$_3$CO-C$_6$H$_4$-C(O)-CH(C$_2$H$_5$)-C$_6$H$_3$(OCH$_3$)(NO$_2$)

9

1. N$_2$H$_4$/Ni
2. Mg(C$_2$H$_5$)Br

H$_3$CO-C$_6$H$_4$-C(OH)-CH(C$_2$H$_5$)-C$_6$H$_3$(OCH$_3$)(NH$_2$) C$_2$H$_5$

8

Δ

10

1. CH$_2$—CH$_2$ O
2. SOCl$_2$

$\rightarrow$

C$_6$H$_3$(OCH$_3$)[N(CH$_2$-CH$_2$Cl)$_2$] ... H$_3$CO-C$_6$H$_4$

11

Fig. 6

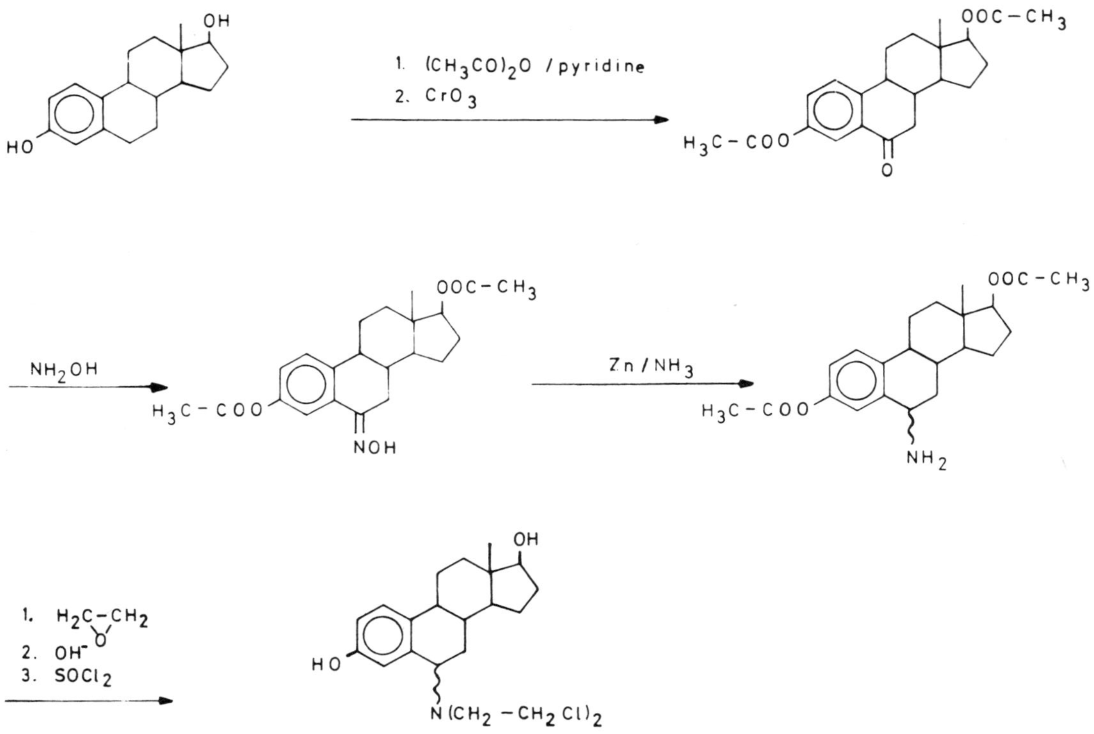

Fig. 7

Toxicological results

The results of acute toxicity testing of some of the alkylating estrogen derivatives are shown in Fig. 8. The compounds were dissolved in dimethylsulphoxide and administered subcutaneously or intraperitoneally. The acute toxicity (DL_{50}) of diethylstilbestrol and the hexestrol derivatives with free hydroxyl groups and two N-mustard groups linked to the carrier was found to be in the same order of 10 to 20 mg/kg body weight. As expected, the toxicity of the estrone derivative with one N-mustard group in 2-position of the steroid ring system with a DL_{50} of 75 mg/kg body weight was lower. However, the corresponding 4-mustard estrone derivative with a DL_{50} of 7 mg/kg body weight was even more toxic than the bifunctional mustard derivatives of diethylstilbestrol or hexestrol. We have no explanation for this surprising result.

Conclusions

The results of the binding studies of the available cytotoxic estrogens clearly show that the free hydroxyl groups of the estrogen carrier cannot be modified without a considerable decrease in receptor affinity. Moreover, linkage of the cytotoxic function to the carrier by esterification may cause a fast hydrolysis of the cytotoxic groups before the compounds reach their target cells. Therefore, a direct connection between, for example, the N atom of a mustard group and the carbon skeleton of the carrier should be favourable. The synthesis of compounds of this type has proved to be difficult, particularly if the hydroxyl groups of the carrier are to be free.

As the hydroxyl groups of the carrier are apparently involved in the binding process at the receptor site, a longer distance between them and the cytotoxic functions should be stereochemically advantageous for receptor affinity.

The aim of this kind of antitumor drug design should be the linkage of cytotoxic groups to suitable carriers in such a manner that receptor affinity is preserved. Even when we succeed in achieving this, another problem will remain, namely the selective and destructive effect of the cytotoxic compounds on the target substrate in the tumor cells. The following types of behaviour of cytotoxic estrogens are conceivable.

1. The cytotoxic groups react with physiological substrates outside the tumor cell.
2. They enter the tumor cells in unchanged form, but are lacking receptor affinity.
3. The unchanged compounds bind to the estrogen receptor but

Acute Toxicity in Mice

	DL 50
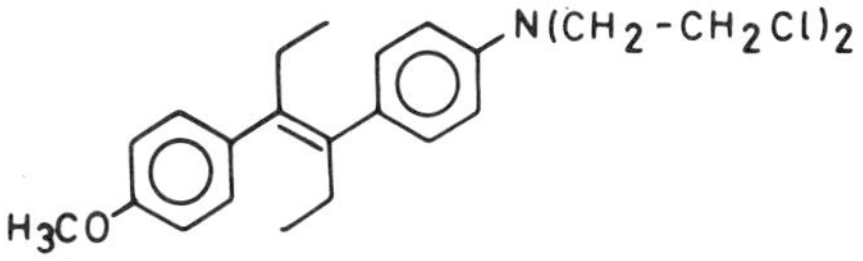	
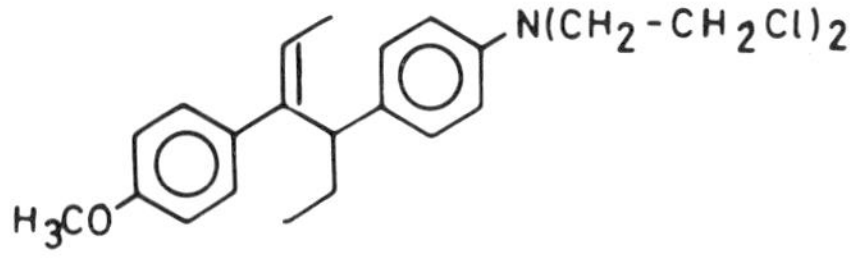	>300 mg/kg s.c.
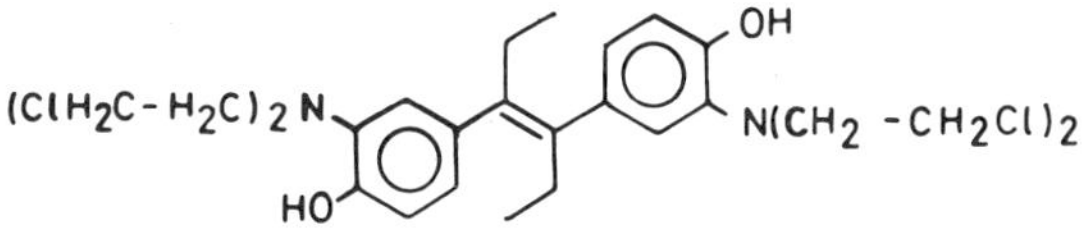	20 mg/kg i.p.
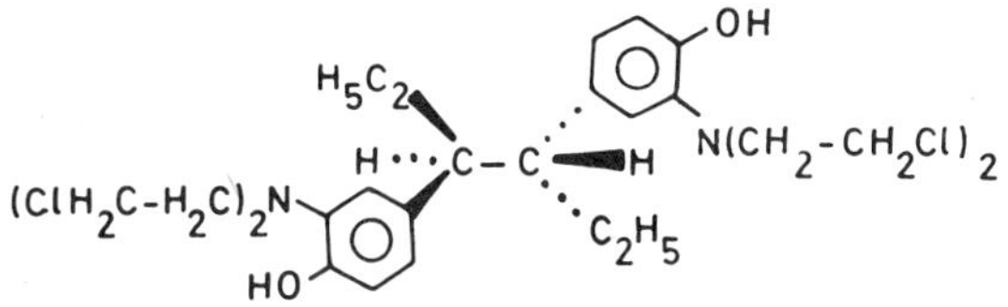	11 mg/kg i.p.
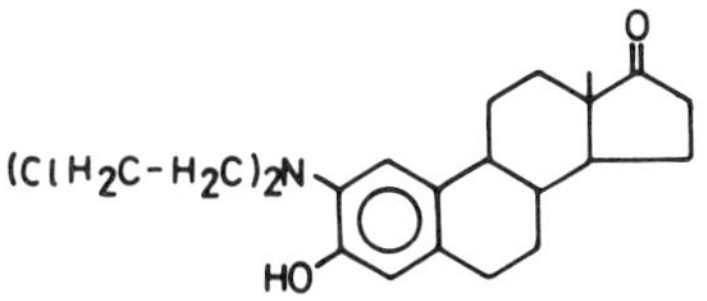	75 mg/kg i.p.
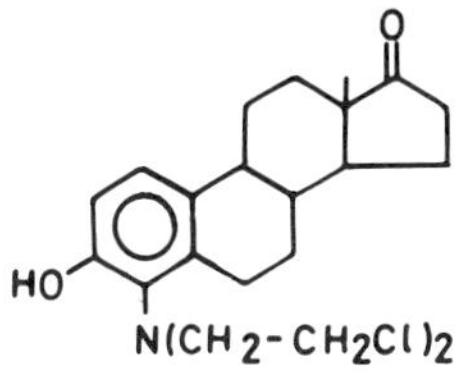	7 mg/kg i.p.

Fig. 8

cannot be transported to the cell nucleus.

4. They are transported to the tumor cell nucleus by the normal hormone transport mechanism but have no intrinsic activity.
5. They act as estrogen hormones by the normal mechanism.

Compounds of type 4 would have the best properties to exert the intended selective action against estrogen-receptor-containing cancer cells. A prerequisite for such compounds is not only a high receptor affinity of the cytotoxic estrogens but also a suitable reactivity of the cytotoxic group itself. With regard to this factor, the variation of the cytotoxic functional groups deserves considerable attention in future synthetic work.

References

Carrol, F. J. et al., *J. med. Chem.* **15**, 1158 (1972)
Clark, E. R., S. R. O'Donnell, *J. Chem. Soc.* **1965**, 6509
Hamacher, H., *Arzneim. Forsch.* **29**, 463 (1979)
Hamacher, H., Brecht, B., Arch. Pharm. Weinheim, *Ger.* **310**, 662 (1977)
Hamacher, H., *ibid.* **311**, 184 (1978)
Larionov, L. F. et al., *Vop. Onkol.* **1968**, 14 (11), 61; *C. A.* **70**, 34726 b (1969).

Discussion

Epstein: Could you tell me how you proceeded when you tried to dehydrate your 3,4-diphenyl-3-hydroxy-hexane?

Hamacher: We tested different conditions. We first tried the thermal way. We performed other trials in acidic conditions but we could not isolate the compound which we wanted.

Epstein: You never tried to get the tosylate and eliminate it in basic conditions?

Hamacher: No, we haven't done this.

Leclercq: With your new compound, with the mustard in position 6, do you believe that you could have the two epimers, the one in position α and the other in position β, or only one?

Hamacher: We are not sure. These investigations are in progress, I don't have the results as yet but I think it is only one compound.

Katzenellenbogen: Why are you interested in the stilbestrol series, rather than the hexestrol series? I think that you could make the mono-substitued hexestrols quite simply by nitration of hexestrol.

Hamacher: We are doing this. We started with diethylstilbestrol because in the first papers published it seemed to have a much higher receptor affinity.

Katzenellenbogen: Is there a tendency of the ortho-N mustards to cyclize onto the phenolic hydroxyl?

Hamacher: There seems to be. When we crystallize these compounds, we see that they are changing, they are discoloring. They are not very stable.

Morgan: The attachment of cytotoxic moieties onto natural estrogens in order to carry the former groups into hormone sensitive cells is intriguing. One continuous controversy with Estracyt is that the cytotoxic group is attached through an ester group which is sensitive to esterases with hydrolysis *in vivo* before entering the cancer cell. Simple 3-methyl ethers of estrone are weakly estrogenic probably as a result of eliminating the hydrogen donating properties of the estrone 3-hydroxyl and its attachment to the natural estrogen receptor.

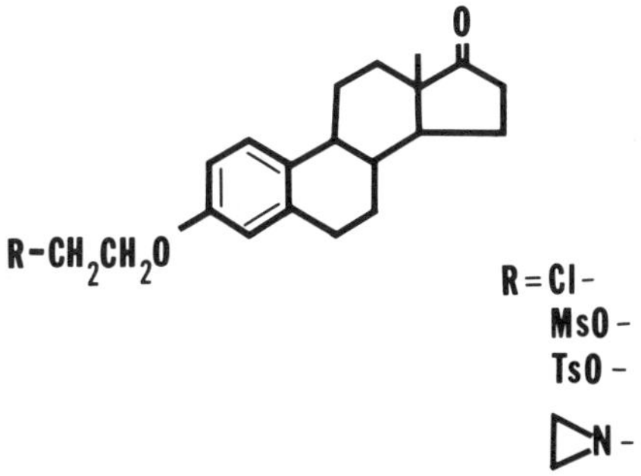

$$R-CH_2CH_2O-$$

$$R = Cl-$$
$$MsO-$$
$$TsO-$$

We have synthesized β-sulfonates of the 3-ethyl ether of estrone - mesyl (Mso) and p-tosyl (Tso). The corresponding chloro- and imine substitutions were also synthesized. Through the electron withdrawing properties of the sulfonates, the ether oxygen appears to have a greater affinity to the estrogen receptor than do simple ethers. In comparison to the binding of estradiol (Estradiol = 100) the relative binding for Mso = 15, Tso = 10 and the Cl and imine < 3 each. Under physiological conditions, the sulfonates are stable for 2 hours but do undergo solvolysis and carbonium ion formation with alkylation properties. The usefulness of the sulfonate group in these cytotoxic compounds is encouraging.

Zeelen: I did not understand your argument on the electronic effect of the mesylate, because the 3-O H function is mainly an H-bridge donor and not an acceptor, so how could the mesylate influence that?

Morgan: When the oxygen interacts with the aromatic ring, there is a positivity that develops on the oxygen, that will allow it to interact with the receptor. A comparison of the binding of a methyl ether with the one of a vinyl ether shows a higher binding of the vinyl ether compound to the receptor. The tosylate was expected to do the same thing without being as reactive as the vinyl ethers. This of course is not in agreement with the H-binding of the free hydroxyl grouping.

Lam: If the estrogen receptor (ER) is involved in the antitumor mechanism of an estrogen-alkylating agent conjugate, an ideal conjugate would be expected to have the following properties:

a) The conjugate should be able to bind to ER. Ideally, the ER-drug complex would be translocated into the nucleus where the alkylating agent would be released to act on the presumed primary target molecule, DNA. If translocation fails to occur, concentrative accumulation may still take place.

b) The alkylating moiety should be linked to the estrogen by a labile bond. Many factors, such as the steric factor, chemical reactivity, physical property, etc., are involved in the interaction of the alkylating agent and the DNA molecule. To design an estrogen-alkylating agent conjugate, one may link the alkylating moiety to different positions on the estrogen by a stable bond, to obtain a compound which is able to react with DNA. However, this approach appears to be impractical not only because of the large number of possible drug-hormone combinations but also because the conditions permitting the conjugate to interact with DNA are unknown. Another approach is to link some known active alkylating moiety to estrogen by a "labile" bond, e.g. ester, amide, disulfide, etc. Enzymatic or chemical cleavage of these bonds *in vivo* would set free the active alkylating moiety which might interact with the target molecule DNA, irrespective of the steroid structure. This approach seems more practical and more likely to produce active antitumor agents.

c) The products formed after the release of the alkylating moiety should have less affinity for the receptor than that of the parent conjugate. Otherwise, the high affinity products would interfere with the binding of the parent conjugate to ER and prevent the selective accumulation of the estrogen-alkylating agent conjugate in cancer cells. We found that an estrogen-nitrosourea conjugate satisfies these three criteria.

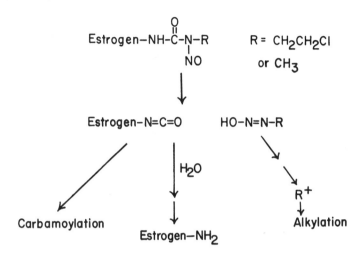

If one or both hydroxyl groups on the estrogen moiety essential for ER binding are retained, the estrogen-nitrosourea conjugate will be expected to have some affinity for ER. Upon decomposition (i.e. activation), the conjugate, like other nitrosoureas, would be expected to generate a chloroethyl or methyl carbonium ion and an isocyanate linked to the estrogen molecule. The reactive carbonium ion will act as the alkylating agent, therefore the position on the estrogen where the nitrosourea moiety is linked will not be a crucial factor in the alkylating reaction. If the nitrosourea decomposes in the cytosol or in the circulation, the estrogen-isocyanate may carbamylate nucleophiles such as proteins or other small molecules with nucleophilic functions. Otherwise, the reaction with water will subsequently form an estrogen-amine. As aliphatic amines are usually protonated at physiological pH, the positive charge on the estrogen-amine may interfere with its binding to ER. All estrogen-amine derivatives we studied have a relative binding affinity at least one order of magnitude lower than that of the corresponding nitrosourea derivative.

We have synthesized several estrogen-nitrosourea conjugates, including estradiol (J. Med. Chem. 22:200, 1979), diethylstilbestrol and other biphenolic derivatives. The apparent binding affinity of 17α- and 17β- substituted estradiol nitrosourea conjugates are about 2%

and 0.2% of that of estradiol, respectively.

Studies of the antitumor activity of these compounds are now in progress.

Könyves: There are two main ways of linking cytostatic agents to steroids; one being the attachment of cytostatic groups directly to one of the carbon atoms of the steroidal skeleton, the other by linking these agents by means of a connection group to the steroids. We selected the second way, contrary to the way which was presented by Hamacher and coworkers (Hamacher), because of the possibility to prepare drugs which can be seen as pro-drugs as far as the steroids are concerned and which can also easily be synthesized as compounds with low reactivity and low general toxicity (Könyves, 1976).

One of the ways to reach this goal is to attach alkylating agents in the form of a carbamate to various steroids. In this type of alkylating agent a mustard part is located in the form of a carbamate in various positions of the steroid skeleton, which can be supposed to be stable *in vivo.*

STEROID CARBAMATES OF THE GENERAL FORMULA:

$$\text{STEROID}-\text{O}-\overset{\overset{\text{O}}{\|}}{\text{C}}-\text{N} \overset{\diagup\text{CH}_2\text{CH}_2\text{Cl}}{\diagdown\text{CH}_2\text{CH}_2\text{Cl}}$$

STEROIDS	AUTHOR	YEAR
1. STEROL	OWEN ET AL.	1956
2. ESTROGENS	NOGRADY ET AL.	1962
	LEO, SWEDEN	1963
	NICULESCU-DUVAZ ET AL.	1967
3. ANDROGENS	CIORANESCU AND RAILEANU	1962
	LEO, SWEDEN	1963
4. GESTOGENS	LEO, SWEDEN	1963
5. CORTICOIDS	LEO, SWEDEN	1963
	RAILEANU AND CIORANESCU	1963

The Table shows the chronological succession of the published N-bis-(2-chloroethyl)carbamates. The first paper in this series by Owen and coworkers (Owen *et al.*, 1956) deals with cholesteryl carbamates. As the table shows, various groups in Canada (Nogrady *et al.*, 1962), Roumania (Cioranescu *et al.*, 1962; Niculescu-Duvaz *et al.*, 1967; Raileanu *et al.*, 1963) and Sweden have been working independently to connect the nor-nitrogen mustard in the form of a carbamate to various steroids.

The carbamate group may be used as a link for other types of cytostatic agents. For instance, as is apparent from Type 2 of Figure 1, if one of the 2-chloroethyl groups of the N-bis (2-chloroethyl)carbamate moiety (Type 1) is replaced by a nitroso group, a steroid N-(2-chloroethyl)-N-nitroso carbamate is obtained. The interest in nitroso carbamates arose already during World War II. Studies showed that the physiological effects of compounds of this type, being carbamates of lower alkanols and phenols, resembled, to some extent, those obtained with mustard gas (Crawford *et al.*, 1943). All these types of compounds were found to be highly toxic (Ross, 1967). In view of this background the following question is posed: Is it possible to decrease the toxicity and introduce antitumor activity by using a steroid hormone as a biological carrier of the N-(2-chloroethyl)-N-nitroso carbamate group by analogy to the steroid-bis-(2-chloroethyl) carbamates? In our research programme we synthesized estrogens, androgens, gestogens, corticosteroids and sterols, where the nitroso chloroethyl carbamates were attached in various positions of the steroidal skeleton (Könyves *et al.*, 1978). Some of the estrogen compounds had an ED 50 about 1 x 0.25 mg per kg without being toxic at a dose of 1 x 1000 mg per kg, when these were tested in the AH130 hepatoma tumor by i.p. administration.

As a result of the screening data obtained in AH130 hepatoma and in L1210 lymphocytic leukaemia by i.p. administration we can make

STEROID CYTOSTATIC CARBAMATES

SYNTHETIZED BY AB LEO RESEARCH LABORATORIES

$$\text{TYPE 1: STEROID-O-}\overset{\overset{\text{O}}{\|}}{\text{C}}\text{-N}\overset{\diagup CH_2CH_2Cl}{\diagdown CH_2CH_2Cl}$$

$$\text{TYPE 2: STEROID-O-}\overset{\overset{\text{O}}{\|}}{\text{C}}\text{-N}\overset{\diagup NO}{\diagdown CH_2CH_2Cl}$$

the following conclusions:
1) The nitroso group is essential for good antitumor activity
2) The halogen atom in the ω -Haloethyl carbamate is essential too for the antitumor activity
3) The halogen should preferably be located in the 2-position of the alkyl group
4) The halogen of the haloethyl group should preferably be chlorine, as bromine gives lower antitumor activity and the fluorine analog shows higher toxicity.

Results in DMBA-induced rat mammary tumors indicate that some of these compounds have good inhibitory effects on the growth of the tumors (Bouveng *et al.,* 1979).

At present we are studying the pharmacokinetic and the toxicological properties of these compounds.

References

Alexander, N. C., Hanock, A. K., Masood, M. B., Peet, B. G., Price, J. J., Turner, R. L., Stone, A., and Ward, J. (1979). *Clin. Radiol.* **30**, 139.

Andersson, L., Edsmyr, F., Jönsson, G., and Könyves, L. (1977). *Recent Results in Cancer Research* **60**, 173. ED. : E. Grundmann and W. Vahlensieck.

Bouveng, R., Ellmann, M., Gunnarsson, P. O., Jensen, G., Liljekvist, J., and Müntzing, J. (1979). *Europ. J. Cancer* **15**, 407.

Cioranescu, E., and Raileanu, D. (1962). *Acad. Rep. Populare Romine, Studii Cercetari Chim.* **10**, 295.

Crawford, B. and Smith, W. W. (1943). *PB Rept.* **140**, 100 (Ref: Chem. Abstr. 54: 17677f (1960).

Groupe Européen du Cancer du Sein. (1969). *Europ. J. Cancer* **5**, 1.

Hamacher, H. refers to the lecture by Hamacher at the present workshop.

Jönson, G., Högberg, B., and Nilsson, T. (1977). *Scand. J. Urol. Nephrol.* **11**, 231.

Könyves, I., and Liljekvist, J. (1976). *Excerpta Medica International Congress Series* **375**, 98.

Könyves, I., Fex, H., Högberg, B., Jensen, G., and Stamvik, A. (1978). *Excerpta Medica International Congress Series* **420**, 303.

Mittelman, A., Shukla, S. K., Welwaart, K. and Murphy, G. P. (1975). *Cancer Chemother. Rep., Part* **1**, 219.

Niculescu-Duvaz, I., Cambanis, A., and Feyns, V. (1967). *Rev. Chim.* **18** (5), 296.

Nogrady, T., Vagi, K. M., and Adamkiewicz, V. W. (1962). *Can. J. Chem.* **40**, 2126.

Owen, L. N., Benn, M. H., and Creighton, A. M. (1956). *British Empire Cancer Campaign* **34**, 448.

Raileanu, D., and Cioranescu, E. (1963). *Acad. Rep. Populare Romine, Studii Cercetari Chim.,* **11** (3-4), 433.

Ross, W. C. J. (1967). *J. Med. Chem.* **10** (1), 108.

16α-IODO-17β-ESTRADIOL: A HIGHLY SPECIFIC RADIOIODINATED PROBE FOR THE ESTROGEN RECEPTOR

RICHARD B. HOCHBERG

Department of Medicine, The Roosevelt Hospital
Department of Biochemistry, College of
Physicians and Surgeons, Columbia University
New York, N.Y. 10019, U.S.A.

Introduction

The synthesis of tritium labeled estradiol of relatively high specific activity in the laboratory of Jensen (1960) led directly to the first demonstration that steroid target organs were capable of concentrating steroid hormones against a blood gradient. Through the use of this tritiated steroid the cytoplasmic estrogen receptor (ER) was then discovered and our understanding of the manner in which hormones exert their effects was forever changed. Even before [^{3}H] estradiol was synthesized attempts had been made to prepare a radioiodine labeled estrogen (Albert, 1949). These attempts were followed by many others (Katzenellenbogen *et al.*, 1975; Counsell *et al.*, 1976; Komai *et al.*, 1977; Katzenellenbogen *et al.*, 1975; Tubis *et al.*, 1967), and while it was possible to synthesize analogs of estrogens labeled with iodine, none of these compounds were useful for studies of binding to the estrogen receptor.

These iodinated compounds were synthesized even though [^{3}H] estradiol was available because of the enormous advantages that a gamma emitter offers over a Beta emitter. γ-Emitters, such as ^{125}I are not only counted more easily and cheaply than β-emitters but the difference in specific activity of ^{125}I, approximately 2,200 Ci/mmole, compared to [^{3}H], about 29 Ci/mmole, or approximately 100 Ci/mM when multiple [^{3}H] atoms are incorporated into a molecule, allows for much more sensitive and precise receptor analyses with ^{125}I. This enormous increase in specific activity and in the energy of the emissions obtained with radioiodine labeled estrogens would allow the facile detection of ER in tissues, especially heterogenous tissues which contain even smaller concentrations of the receptor than the minute amounts present in classical target organs. Thus, not only are more sensitive chemical analyses possible but other techniques, such as the detection of ER by autoradiographic studies could be shortened from months or years to weeks or even days. Through the use of isotopes that can be spectrally differentiated, such as ^{125}I and ^{131}I, experiments on receptor turnover and synthesis can be performed directly. Furthermore, radioiodine labeled estrogens could play an important clinical role. Through the use of radioimaging equipment, ^{123}I or ^{131}I labeled estrogens could be used *in vivo* for visualizing and detecting estrogen responsive tumors or metastases. The high energies of the γ and β emissions of an ^{131}I labeled estrogen might have utility as a therapeutic agent for the destruction of such cancers.

As delineated by Katzenellenbogen *et al.* (1975) there are several criteria necessary for an iodinated steroid to be useful for receptor studies: it must bind with high affinity to the receptor; it must not bind excessively to high capacity, low affinity proteins and the linkage of the iodine atom must be both chemically and metabolically stable. There are further constraints: the half-life limitations of the various isotopes of iodine require that the procedure for synthesis should not be time consuming and the procedure should be capable of producing steroids labeled with a high specific activity. This report describes a radioiodine labeled estrogen, 16α-[^{125}I]iodo-17β-estradiol (^{125}I-E$_2$) that meets all of these requirements (Korenman, 1969) (Fig. 1). Estradiol was labeled at carbon 16 because it is known that estriol like estradiol binds to the ER (Korenman, 1969; Ruh *et al.*, 1973) and it seemed reasonable that substitution at this position would not block this interaction. Recently, it has also been shown that various C-16 iodinated steroidal estrogens are

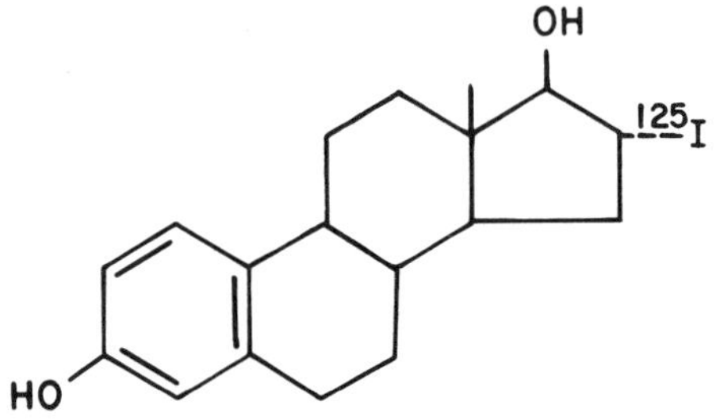

Fig. 1: 16α[^{125}I] iodo-17β-estradiol

potent inhibitors of the binding of $[^3H]E_2$ to ER (Arunchalam *et al.*, 1979).

Synthesis

The synthetic route used to synthesize ^{125}I-E_2 is the exchange of 16β-bromoestradiol (16Br-E_2) with $Na^{125}I$. The starting material, 16Br-E_2 was synthesized by bromination of the enoldiacetate of estrone and then reduction of the resulting 16α-bromoestrone with $NaBH_4$ (Hochberg, 1979). This procedure for synthesizing ^{125}I-E_2 has several distinct advantages. Most importantly, the reaction leads to epimerization at C-16, and the resulting radioactive 16α-iodo compound can be readily separated from the 16β-bromo substrate by a variety of chromatographic techniques. Theoretically carrier free material can be obtained, even in the presence of the large excess of Br-E_2 necessary for the halogen exchange reaction. Once the stable Br-E_2 is synthesized enough material is obtained in even small reactions for thousands of iodinations. The exchange procedure is simple and requires only commercially available radioiodine in the form of NaI. In addition it is adaptable to any of the isotopes of iodine.

The tracer, ^{125}I-E_2 is synthesized by incubating 10 μg of Br-E_2 with 1-2 mCi of carrier free $Na^{125}I$ in 2-butanone at 70° overnight. The next morning the reaction mixture is extracted and chromatographed on a small column of silica gel (Hochberg, 1979). In this system the tracer I-E_2 separates cleanly from the Br-E_2 reactant. Run under nitrogen pressure this chromatograph takes 4 hours. In addition, the material is chromatographed by high pressure chromatography (HPLC) (Fig. 2). In this system the iodinated product is purified in less than 15 minutes. Consequently the reaction and purification is completed in less than one working day. The yield of I-E_2 usually approximates 50% of the radioiodine incubated. The specific activity of the product is determined through the use of a sensitive UV detector (280 nm) coupled to the HPLC. While the Na ^{125}I is carrier free, the iodinated ligand has not been synthesized in carrier free form. Although I-E_2 with a specific activity of approximately 1200-1400 Ci/mmol is now regularly synthesized, initial efforts produced material of 50-150 Ci/mmol, and some of the experiments described are with this lower specific acitvity ligand. This decrease from theoretical specific activity was caused by traces of 16α-bromoestradiol present in the 16Br-E_2 substrate and because some of the α-bromo analog is also formed through epimerization by an impurity in the radioiodine. The 16α-bromoestradiol is not readily separated from I-E_2 by chromatography.

The identity of ^{125}I-E$_2$ was ascertained by reverse isotope dilution and crystallization with authentic 16α-iodoestradiol. The ^{125}I labeled estrogen is stable and shows little sign of decomposition after weeks of storage at 4°.

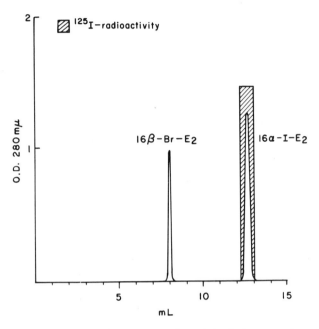

Fig. 2: High pressure liquid chromatography of the halogen exchange reaction (Na^{125}I and 16β - bromoestradiol). Chromatography was performed on a Lichrosorb Diol column (250 x 4.6 mm), Merck Co., with methylene chloride at a flow rate of 1 ml min. Another chromatogram of the non-radioactive substrate and product is superimposed.

In Vivo Experiments

In order to determine if I-E$_2$ would be recognized as an estrogen by target tissues, two experiments were performed. First, various amounts of non-radioactive I-E$_2$ were injected into immature rats and its estrogenic potency was compared to E$_2$ in a uterotrophic assay. The results shown in Fig. 3 demonstrate that I-E$_2$ causes a dramatic increase in the weight of the uterus. In this assay it has approximately 1/4 to 1/5 the effect of E$_2$, or 4 to 5 times that of estrone (Emmens, 1962). Obviously I-E$_2$ is a very potent estrogen. The second experiment was designed to determine if the uterus would concentrate the iodinated estrogen (Hochberg, 1979). Mature castrated female rats were injected with 0.5 μCi of ^{125}I-E$_2$ (< 100 Ci/mmol) and after 6 hours the amount of radioactivity incorporated into a

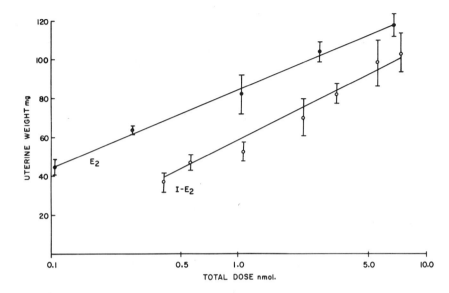

Fig. 3: Bioassay of 16α-iodoestradiol. Immature female rats were injected for three consecutive days with either E_2 or 16α -I-E_2 dissolved in sesame oil. On the fourth day the uteri were removed and weighed.

TABLE I

In vivo tissue uptake of 16α-^{125}I-estradiol

Tissue	CPM/100 mg tissue		% ether extractable
		+DES	
Uterus	313 ± 150	73 ± 8	>90
Liver	446 ± 184	425 ± 105	10 - 15
Kidney	73 ± 33	75 ± 20	
Serum	69 ± 11	68 ± 6	
Lung	47 ± 23	56 ± 11	
Muscle	33 ± 23	18 ± 12	
Heart	23 ± 5	26 ± 7	
Thyroid*	1839 ± 809	2287 ± 805	0 - 1

In vitro Uptake of 16α- ^{125}I-E_2. Castrated female rats were injected subcutaneously with 0.5uCi of 16α-[125] I-E_2. Another group of rats received 5 mg of DES 20 minutes prior to the administration of the tracer. Six hours later the animals were sacrificed and the organs were weighed and counted. All value are ± S.D.. * the radioactivity in the thyroid is per the entire organ. (From Hochberg *et al.*, 1979).

variety of tissues was measured. The data in Table I shows that on a weight basis the amount of radioactivity in the uterus was greater than any other tissue with the exception of the liver and the thyroid. When 5 μg of diethylstilbesterol (DES) was injected into the rats 20 minutes before the administration of the tracer the only organ which showed a decrease in the uptake of radioactivity was the uterus. This competition by the non-steroidal estrogen DES demonstrates the specificity of the uterine uptake. Furthermore, when the uterus, liver and thyroid were extracted and then partioned between ether and aqueous $NaHCO_3$, only the isotope extracted from the uterus was found in the ether. When the radioactivity in the ether extract from the uterus was characterized by HPLC it proved to be almost entirely unchanged $^{125}I\text{-}E_2$. Thus, of all the tissues examined only the uterus concentrated unmetabolized $I\text{-}E_2$. The radioactivity in the thyroid is probably due to uptake of $[^{125}I]$ iodide liberated from $I\text{-}E_2$, and it is equivalent to only 0.2% of the injected dose.

Receptor Studies

The most likely explanation for both the concentration of $I\text{-}E_2$ in

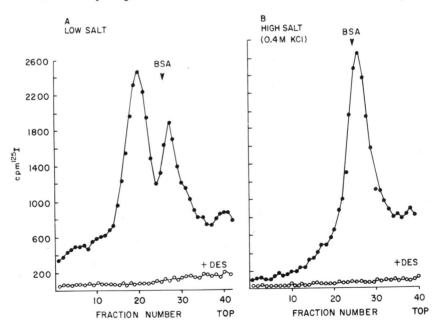

Fig. 4: Gradient centrifugation of $16\alpha\text{-}^{125}I\text{-}E_2$ bound to the estrogen receptor of rat uterine cytosol (From Hochberg *et al.* 1979).

the uterus and for its estrogenicity is that I-E$_2$ is readily bound by the estrogen receptor and this presumption was tested in several experiments. Figure 4 shows a density gradient centrifugation of uterine cytosol which had been incubated with ^{125}I-E$_2$. As would be expected for the estrogen reception in low ionic strength buffer, radioactive peaks with mobilities of 8S and 4S are apparent (Fig. 4A). In 0.4M KCl (Fig. 4B) only the 4S peak appears. A 100 molar excess of DES efficiently displaces the iodinated tracer from both the 8S and 4S peak.

This demonstration that I-E$_2$ was bound to the ER provided impetus for further experiments that measured the affinity of ER for this iodinated ligand. Figure 5 shows the results of an incubation of [125]

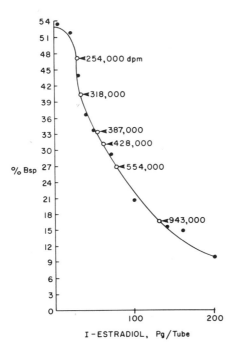

Fig. 5: The determination of the specific activity of 16α-^{125}I-E2. Filled circles: a trace of 16α-^{125}I-E$_2$ (61,000dpm) combined with varying amounts of 16α-iodoestradiol were incubated with calf uterine cytosol and the specifically bound steroid was determined. Opened circles o: varying amounts of 16α-^{125}I-E$_2$ were simultaneously analyzed. The specifically bound radioactivity of 16α-^{125}I-E$_2$ alone was then fitted to the curve obtained with the cold steroid and a specific activity of 1,310 Ci/mmole was obtained. (See Roulston, 1979 for details of the method).

130   R.B. Hochberg

I-E$_2$ with calf uterine cytosol. The bound steroid was separated by charcoal adsorbtion. This figure compares the specific binding of various amounts of ^{125}I-E$_2$ alone to the binding of a trace amount of ^{125}I-E$_2$ combined with increasing concentrations of non-radioactive I-E$_2$. Non-specific binding was again determined with an excess

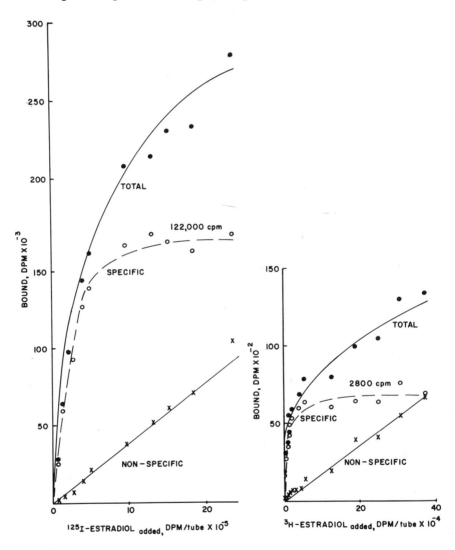

Fig. 6: Saturation analysis of the binding of 16α-^{125}I-E$_2$ (1310 Ci/mmole and ^{3}H-E$_2$ (43 Ci/mmole) to calf uterine cytosol.

of DES and was subtracted from the total bound. By overlapping and comparing these 2 curves the specific activity of the iodinated ligand can be obtained (Roulston, 1979). The specific experiment illustrated in fig 5 provided a specific activity of ^{125}I-E$_2$ of 1310 Ci/mmole which compares well with the value of 1250 Ci/mmole obtained by UV adsorbtion at 280 nm on the HPLC.

The enormous increase in sensitivity of ER binding assays which this tracer provides is apparent in Fig. 6 which shows the saturation analysis curve obtained with this ^{125}I-E$_2$ and a comparison with [^{3}H]E$_2$ (43 Ci/mmole). Both assays were performed simultaneously. The specifically bound radioactivity (in terms of counts per minute) of the iodinated ligand, 122,000 cpm, was almost 45 times greater

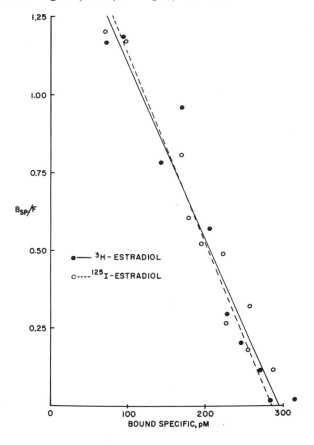

Fig. 7: Scatchard analysis of the binding of 16α-^{125}[I]-E$_2$ and [^{3}H]E$_2$ to calf uterine cytosol. data was obtained from figure 5.

than that of $[^3H]E_2$, 2,800 cpm. When the data in Fig. 6 was plotted in its more usual form, as described by Scatchard (1949), two other important aspects are seen (Fig. 7). The K_d, calculated from the slope of the lines, is identical for the ^3H (1.5 x $10^{-10}M/L$) and ^{125}I (1.4 x $10^{-10}M/L$) labeled steroids. In addition the number of binding sites obtained from the intercept of those lines with the abscissa are also identical for both ligands.

The fact that $I-E_2$ binds to the ER with the same K_d and to the same number of binding sites as E_2 but with an enormous increase in the amount of radioactivity bound, demonstrates that $I-E_2$ is an excellent ligand for estrogen receptor analyses. Furthermore, the non-specific binding of $I-E_2$ is slightly less than that of $[^3H]E_2$ (Fig. 6) which would also help increase the accuracy of an ER assay. When the specificity of this interaction was determined by measuring the binding of $[^3H]$ and $[^{125}I]E_2$ in the presence of several steroids, only estrogenic compounds interfered with the binding of both ligands (Hochberg, et al., 1979). As would be expected from the association constants, $I-E_2$ and E_2 were equal in displacing both radioactive ligands from the ER. Androgens, progestins and corticoids had no effect.

MCF-7 Cells in Culture

The fact that $I-E_2$ has the same affinity for the receptor when compared to E_2 might be surprising in light of the bioassay which showed $I-E_2$ to be considerably less potent than E_2. However, the smaller uteropic effect of $I-E_2$ in vivo when compared to E_2, could reflect a different metabolic fate or clearance of the iodinated steroid or perhaps some post receptor effect. That it is the former is clear clear from some in vitro experiments performed on the estrogen dependent MCF-7 human breast tumor grown in culture (Lippman, 1979). In this system $I-E_2$ and E_2 are equipotent in inducing the progesterone receptor, increasing thymidine incorporation and in promoting growth. In this in vitro model, which is not subject to the metabolic uncertainties of the in vivo assay, $I-E_2$ produced the same estrogenic effects as E_2.

It was demonstrated that these cellular events were probably mediated by a direct receptor mechanism. Both $[^3H]$ and $[^{125}I]E_2$ were incubated with intact MCF-7 cells at 0° and 37° (Fig. 8). At 0° most of the radioactivity was found in the cytoplasmic receptor fraction and very little in the nucleus. However, at 37° it is apparent that the receptor bound with either ligand had translocated into the nucleus. It was also found with MCF-7 cells that $^{125}I-E_2$ could be used in a

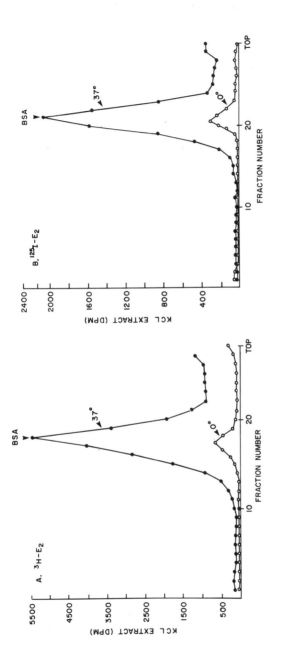

Fig. 8: Nuclear translocation of MCF-7 ER. MCF-7 cells were incubated with both ^3H-E_2 and ^{125}I-E_2 (approx. same specific activity) at 0°; open circles, 0 and at 37°; closed circles, ●. Nuclear pellets were isolated and 0.4M KCl extract were centrifuged on a sucrose gradient. BSA: internal standard of ^{14}C bovine serum albumin.

nuclear exchange assay to measure ER which had been translocated into the nucleus with E_2. The values for ER present in the nucleus in this experiment were the same for $^{125}I\text{-}E_2$ and $[^3H]E_2$ (Lippman, 1979).

Human Breast Tumors

As was demonstrated in the calf uterus, the non-specific binding of I-E_2 was lower than that of E_2. However, in human breast tumors a serum protein contaminant, testosterone-estradiol binding globulin (TeBG) which binds E_2 can complicate ER analysis, and produce false positives. When the binding of I-E_2 to TeBG was determined in human pregnancy plasma, it was found that the iodinated steroid was not a ligand for this protein (Hochberg, 1979). Thus the complication of TeBG contamination in human samples can be neglected in ER studies when I-E_2 is used in such determinations. The utility of I-E_2 for measuring ER in human breast cancers was examined directly. In this experiment four human tumors (supplied by Dr.J.Wittliff), two were ER- and two were ER+, were analyzed for ER with both $[^3H]$ and ^{125}I-E_2. The results shown in Table II reveal that the same number of binding sites were found (within experimental error) with both radioactive steroids.

TABLE II

Estrogen receptor content of human breast tumors

Tumor	ER (femtomoles/mg Protein)	
	$16\alpha\text{-}^{125}I\text{-}E_2$	$^3H\text{-}E_2$
126	72	64
124	24	33
101	$\lhd$	$\lhd$
116	$\lhd$	$\lhd$

Cystosol were analyzed for ER with both $16\alpha\text{-}^{125}I\text{-}E_2$ (1200 CI/mmole) and $[^3H]E_2$ (92 Ci/mmole).

From this data it is clear that I-E_2 can be used to monitor the ER in human breast tumors. To date ^{125}I-E_2 has been tested in comparative experiments with $[^3H]E_2$ for binding to ER in the following tissues: rat and bovine uterus, human breast tumors, MCF-7 cell line, rat hypothalamus and pituitary. (The two latter tissues by Dr.E. Peck, personal communication). In all cases, the binding constants and the number of binding sites for the two steroids were found to be identical.

External Localization of ^{131}I-E$_2$

Since the *in vivo* experiment in the rat had shown that ^{125}I-E$_2$ was concentrated in the uterus, and the *in vitro* experiments revealed that this iodinated estrogen was bound with a high association constant to the ER, it seemed likely that this compound labeled with ^{123}I or ^{131}I could be used as an imaging agent for the external detection of ER containing tumors in patients. To this end a preliminary experiment was performed in order to determine whether an ER containing organ, in this case the uterus, could be imaged with ^{131}I-E$_2$. The tra-

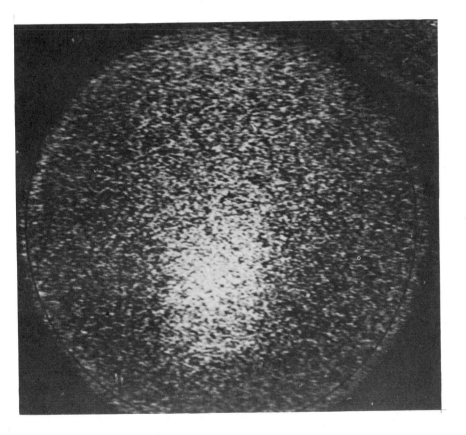

Fig. 9: External localization of squirrel monkey uterus through the use of 16α-^{131}I-E$_2$. γ-rays were detected with an Anger Camera and a pinhole collimator.

cer ^{131}I-E$_2$ was synthesized exactly as described for ^{125}I-E$_2$ with the exception that Na^{131}I was used for the exchange. The subject, a squirrel monkey (Saimari Sciureus), weighing 1.5 kilograms, was ovarietomized 2 weeks before the start of the experiment and an estradiol containing Silastic implant was placed subcutaneously in her back. The implant was removed 24 hours before the intravenous injection of 200 uCi of the tracer dissolved in saline. The animal was scanned constantly with a pin-hole collimator and uptake of the tracer in the liver could be seen immediately. Within 1 of 2 hours radioactivity could be detected in the suprapubic region, but when the bladder was aspirated and washed, 3.8 uCi of radioactivity was found in the urine. At this point the amount of radioactivity detected by the scanner was greatly reduced but another region of radioactivity immediately adjacent to the bladder then became apparent. Since this region of radioactivity (Fig. 9) was present in the correct anatomical location, and because further aspiration and washing of the bladder did not reduce the intensity of the radiation, it appears that the uterus was imaged. These results indicate that ^{123}I-E$_2$ or ^{131}I-E$_2$ might be useful as radioimaging agents for the detection of ER containing cancers.

Acknowledgement

Much of this work was done in collaboration with Dr. William Rosner, Columbia University and Dr. Marc E. Lippman, National Institutes of Health (USA). This work was supported in part by NIH grants: KO4-CA00174 and ROI-CA241512 and by a grant from the Orentreich Foundation.

References

Albert, S., Heard, R.D.H., Leblond, C.P. and Saffron, J. (1949). *J. Biol. Chem.* **177.**

Arunchalam, T., Longcope, C., and Caspi, E. (1979). *J. Biol. Chem.* **254,** 5900.

Counsell, R.E., Buswink, A., Korn, N., Ranade, V., and Yu, T. (1976). *In* "Steroid Hormone Action and Cancer" (K.M. Menon and J.R. Rell, eds.), p. 107. Plenum Press, New York.

Emmens, C.W. (1962). *In* "Methods in Hormone Research" Vol II (R.I. Dorfman, ed.), p. 59. Academic Press, New York.

Hochberg, R.B. (1979). *Science* **205,** 1138.

Hochberg, R.B., and Rosner, W. (1979). (Submitted for Publication).

Jensen, H.I., and Jacobson, H.I. (1960). *In* "Biologic Activities of Steroids in Relation to Cancer" (G.Pincus and E.P. Vollmer. eds.), p. 161. Academic Press, New York.

Katzenellenbogen, J.A., and Hsiung, H.M. (1975). *Biochem.* **14,** 1736.

Katzenellenbogen, J.A., Hsiung, H.M., Carlson, K.E., McGuire, W.L., Kraay, R.J. and Katzenellenbogen, B.S. (1975) *Biochem,* **14**, 1742.

Komai, T., Eckelman, W.C., Jonsonbough, R.E., Mazaitis, A., Kubota, H., and Reba, R.C. (1977). *J.Nucl. Med.* **18**, 360.

Korenman, S.G. (1969). *Steroids,* **13**, 163.

Lippman, M.E., and Hochberg, R.B. (1979). In Preparation.

Roulston, J.E. (1979). *Ann. Clin. Biochem.* **16**, 26.

Ruh, T.S., Katzenellenbogen, B.S., Katzenellenbogen, J.A., and Gorski, J., (1973). *Endocrionol.* **92**, 125.

Scatchard, G. (1949). *Ann NY Acad. Sci,* **51**, 660.

Tubis, M., Endrow, J.S., and Blahd, W.H. (1967). *Nucl. Med.,* **6**, 184.

Discussion

Symes: Can you make some comments on your last picture? (Fig. 9)

Hochberg: This is a picture of the liver. Actually when we allow very few counts to accumulate, you can easily detect the lobes of the liver. I think it is clear that the darkest zone is the liver. The liver is extremely hot in comparison to the other tissues. After about one hour we started to see an accumulation of radioactivity in an area which we thought was the uterus, but it turned out to be the bladder. When we aspirated the bladder and washed it, almost all radioactivity disappeared. After a much longer time we were able to pick up another area which did not disappear upon reaspirating and washing the bladder. We felt that this was the uterus.

Katzenellenbogen: What is happening to the intestinal radioactivity?

Hochberg: You can see the intestinal radioactivity very clearly. In the early parts of the experiment the radioactivity accumulates in the liver. Consecutively it gets into the gall bladder and starts coming down the intestine. Within 3 to 4 hours the radioactivity there is still very high. After some time you can actually watch it coming down the intestinal tract so that by the next day most of the radioactivity is localized in the bowel.

Griffiths: Do the 16α-bromo and the 16α-chloro compounds bind as well as the 16α-iodo?

Hochberg: Well I don't know about the chloro, but the bromo binds almost the same way.

Van Lier: Did you know the receptor concentration in the uterus at the time of the experiment?

Hochberg: No. We gave the animal a large amount of estradiol to build up the receptor concentration in the uterus. The dose of estrogen that we gave was a normal dose for a rhesus monkey. The rhesus monkey weighs about ten times as much as the squirrel monkey we used. We removed the implant so that the estradiol level fell basically to zero by the time we ran the experiment, which was a little less than 24 hours later. So I can't answer your question because we didn't sacrifice the animal for this experiment.

Morgan: Have you used the iodo compound in animals with tumors like DMBA tumors?

Hochberg: No we haven't yet. We have done it with I^{125} concentrates. We haven't done it with I^{131} because we have been told that we were going to get lousy pictures. Everybody tells us that I^{131} is the wrong isotope to use and we are now concentrating our efforts on making I^{123} labeled estradiol which is a better agent for imaging and in addition it has a much shorter half life, so we would be able to give it in very large amounts to patients when we are at that point. Right now we have stopped work on I^{131} for this particular type of experiment, although we are still using it for other experiments that I have indicated. When we have the I^{123} compound we'll start these experiments up again.

Katzenellenbogen: So you did I^{125} uptake into the mammary tumors of the DMBA rats. What sort of selectivity did you see?

Hochberg: It is not taken up by mammary tissue as well as by the uterus.

Katzenellenbogen: Did you see the thyroid gland in the monkey?

Hochberg: That is interesting. The first experiment we used a blocking agent and we gave the animal KI because I didn't want the thyroid to pick up radioactivity. The second experiment I forgot to do it, and we didn't get a picture of the thyroid. There was very little radioactivity in the thyroid.

Wittliff: Just a problem that I think those of us who work with titration curves and are using the ligand you synthesized, should be really aware of, is the incredible amount of radioactivity you are using with a reagent that has 1500-200 Curies/mmole. In some of the universities it may be prohibited by the health department.

Hochberg: Obviously you don't have to use material that is very hot.

Wittliff: That is right, but what is commercially available now has a specific activity of 2000 a 200 Curies/mmole. What specific activity are you using?

Hochberg: About 200 Curies/mmole.

Wittliff: I am saying that we should be very careful in using that high specific activity material unless we are going to dilute the receptor and that is dangerous.

Hochberg: That is right, because if you dilute the receptor too much you are running into problems. Indeed upon dilution ligand and receptor don't find each other very well. You get an apparent decrease in receptor concentration which in reality is not taking place. The receptor seems to be less stable under those conditions.

Wittliff: That's why the 200 Curies/mmole reagent seems better to me for routine use. Don't you agree?

Hochberg: Yes, for routine use definitely, but there are very good uses for material with a high specific activity.

Wittliff: Just a comment about a particular type of tumor where this might really help inflammatory carcinoma of the breast, and where histologically you see very few deposits of ligand cells. If you look in the literature and, looking at our own experience with a few inflammatory carcinomas, virtually all of these are negative for estrogen receptor content. I was wondering, whether you have thought about using the reagent in such a way that it could be perfused right before a mastectomy and then take a picture of the mastectomy specimen.

Hochberg: I have been giving a lot of thought to things like that. I was hoping that we could use the I^{125} labeled substance *in vitro*, so that you don't have to make a cytosol preparation.

Some laboratories that don't have ultra centrifuges and things like that could work with the I^{125} labeled material by making radiographic studies for example. However the non-specific binding of this compound and the tritiated estradiol under the condition of cell slices and pieces of tumor are really enormous.

A better use for the high specific activity compound would be to look for a nuclear uptake. If one could localize the radioactivity in the area of the nucleus this would give us a specific indication of micro populations of receptor positive tumors.

Katzenellenbogen: You mentioned that this compound shows lower non-specific binding than estradiol. But these are experiments in which you don't have an equilibrium situation.

Hochberg: Yes, maybe there is some non-specific binding, but this compound doesn't bind to TeBG, at least not in the monkey. The clearance as far as we can see, is very rapid into the liver. Knowing that the halflife is somewhat around 10 min. or less, clearance is very rapid.

Katzenellenbogen: Your low salt sucrose gradients show the 4S peak which is competitive with DES. Do you think that this is receptor, or do you think that this is material which is falling off from the 8S peak and is being bound to albumin or something else?
   That is the sort of thing people have seen with rapidly dissociating estrogens such as tamoxifen.

Hochberg: Everyone of our experiments that we did was done with a control of tritiated estradiol. Every experiment was superimposable in that respect. Whatever we saw with tritiated estradiol in terms of 4S peak was present with the iodinated steroid.

Katzenellenbogen: When you see the 8S peak with tritiated estradiol, is that displaceable?

Hochberg: Yes.

Wittliff: Was that experiment done with rat uterus?

Hochberg: Yes. Dr. Sherman suggested to me that what we were seeing was a proteolysis of the receptor.

PANEL DISCUSSION

Van Lier. We all know that it is important to have a good interaction between the steroid and the receptor, meaning that the bulky group must be as far away from the estrogen as possible. I wonder if you care to discuss the possibilities of what kind of spacers to use or what type of reagent one could think of to put in between the cytotoxic agent and the steroid.

Blickenstaff: One could use methylenediamine. We have considered using several polymethylenediamines to get different chain lengths. But we haven't done it yet.

Zeelen: What is the reason to have two polar groups in it?

Blickenstaff: Chemically, just to make binding. To facilitate the synthesis.

Zeelen: But you pay for it.

Katzenellenbogen: I think we are hearing a suggestion of keeping things as hydrophobic as possible.

Zeelen: Right.

Hochberg: Do you think it is possible if you have to give up something, like hydrophobicity, to counteract it somewhere else in the molecule by putting in another hydrophobic group?

Zeelen: That's indeed one of the possibilities.

Blickenstaff: What is the largest group that has been attached at 17α in estradiol without losing the high binding affinity for the estrogen receptor?

Katzenellenbogen. One of the compounds prepared for affinity chromatography had a very long hydrocarbon chain attached at position 17α.

Zeelen: But the affinity, if I remember well, was down to the range of 5%.

Katzenellenbogen: What is the cytotoxic dose per cell, and for any particular cytotoxic agent we choose can one through a receptor mediated process deliver a cytotoxic dose? This is the question that I asked at the NIH workshop two years ago and it was apparent that no one had really thought about this very much. I also forgot about it until a couple of weeks ago. Then I started calling up some people who might have answers and come up with some numbers. Let me just show the data.

CYTOTOXIC DOSE IN MOLECULES OF CYTOTOXIC AGENT PER CELL

1. Equilibrium model	600,000 (60 x excess over the receptor concentration of 10,000 molecules per cell).
2. DNA-binding model	300,000 (30 x excess).
3. Vinca alkaloids	100,000
4. Methotrexate	144,000,000.
5. FUdR	180,000 - 720,000.
6. Bleomycin	60,000,000.

One thing I think we should point out, is the fact that most of the reagents we have seen, have been ones where the cytotoxic agent is a DNA alkylator. I think this has to do with the fact that we know that estrogens concentrate in the nucleus and perhaps one then tends to think of cytotoxic agents which act on DNA. The Vindecine analogues are a notable exception to that. We know that there are about 10,000 receptor molecules in a receptor-rich cell. A typical cell has a volume of about 100 μm^3. This is probably an underestimate. Most human cells are probably around 3000 μm^3. If one assumes, say in a cell culture experiment, that the cytotoxic agent is active around μmolar concentration and this equivalent concentration is within the medium and within the cell, then just simply by this equilibrium volume calculation the cell would contain 600,000 molecules of cytotoxic agent. This would be a 30-60 fold excess over the receptor concentration. Now this of course is modified by a transport system which may actually cause selective accumulation of the cytotoxic agent in the cell.

The DNA binding model. I got these numbers from someone who said he had done some experiments with actinomycin D and thought it would be true for adriamycin also. At cytotoxic concentration there was about 1 molecule bound per 10^4 base pairs. A human genome has about 2.9 billion base pairs which means that one needs 300,000 molecules per cell as a cytotoxic dose. Again a large excess over available receptor.

The Vinca alkaloids. This is a guess. I don't know what that is based on. I think it is based on some microtubular binding.

Methotrexate. Which does not have DNA as target, but presumably dihydrofolate reductase. One can calculate for the most sensitive cells that there are 144,000,000 molecules of dihydrofolate reductase. Presumably a large fraction of these have to be occupied by methotrexate in order to get the cytotoxic effect. This is a very large excess over receptor.

FUdR: Folium synthetase which is the target for FUdR is present at a concentration of 180,000 - 720,000 molecules per cell.

Bleomycin: The killing concentration is 0.15 mg/ml, which means 60,000,000 molecules per cell.

What we really need if we are going to build nitrosocarbamates, nitrosoureas, nitrogen mustards, is the corresponding measure for these compounds. I don't have any idea of what it is. I suspect it takes more molecules of a cytotoxic agent to kill the cell than there are receptors. However the receptor may in fact act as a transport system in which case it could deliver a quantity that would exceed its capacity. At least if things come off the receptor and react with DNA. This may be a crucial thing to the receptor because it concentrates cytotoxic action within the nucleus or perhaps even within a single site of the nucleus. One could achieve a high local concentration which could lead to cytotoxicity at lower doses. The question of receptor inactivation by these compounds is one we will talk about tomorrow.

To extend the cytotoxicity argument I just want to remind people that there are some exceptionally toxic compounds, which are toxic by a catalytic process, for example diphteria toxin, which is a large protein. Its toxic effect is a catalytic one, where it uses NAD to modify a protein involved in the translocase, and perhaps just a few molecules of this catalytic compound can kill a cell. Colicins, which act on Coli, form ion channels and have DNAse and RNAse activity and one molecule per cell can kill it.

I think we should keep in mind this question of the cytotoxic dose per cell relative to the capacity of the system which we are asking to deliver it. I think cell culture experiments are probably the ones that can give us the most quantitative data. Simple experiments with C^{14} labeled mustard can give us the answer on the number of hits to DNA to kill. I think people who are designing agents like this might want to do these experiments before they spend a lot of time making agents that may not have potential for receptormediated cytotoxicity.

BIOLOGICAL AND ANTINEOPLASTIC EFFECTS

ESTABLISHMENT OF UNIFORMITY IN STEROID RECEPTOR DETERMINATIONS USED IN CLINICAL STUDIES AND DRUG SCREENING PROGRAMS

J. L. WITTLIFF, S. A. WIEHLE, J. P. SANDOZ, B. FISCHER
and J. R. DURANT

Department of Biochemistry, University of Louisville, Kentucky, USA

The concept underlying endocrine therapy is that certain tumors have retained the cellular mechanism to respond to the same hormonal stimuli as their normal progenitor cells. Only recently it was demonstrated that the presence of estrogen receptors provide a molecular basis for the distinction between human breast carcinomas that are responsive to administrative hormonal therapy or to endocrine organ ablative surgery and those which are not (Jensen *et al.*, 1971; McGuire *et al.*, 1975; Wittliff, 1974 & 1978).

Methods of analyses

Steroid receptors have been estimated in a variety of hormone target organs using methods ranging from administration *in vivo* of labeled steroid to procedures *in vitro* (Wittliff, 1975). Two methods have proven useful for the determination of estrogen and progesterone receptors in human breast carcinomas by the clinical chemist. The most commonly employed of these is the titration procedure (Fig. 1) which utilizes dextran-coated charcoal to remove the unbound steroid from that associated with the intracellular receptor and provides a measure of the binding capacity and the affinity. Usually binding capacity is expressed as femtomoles of ^{3}H-labeled steroid bound per mg cytosol protein. It is accepted generally that less than 3 fmol/mg cytosol protein represents a quantity of estrogen binding sites usually correlated with the lack of response of a breast cancer patient given endocrine therapy (McGuire *et al.*, 1975; Raynaud, 1977). Although there is a "borderline" range of values from 3 to 10 fmol/mg cytosol protein,

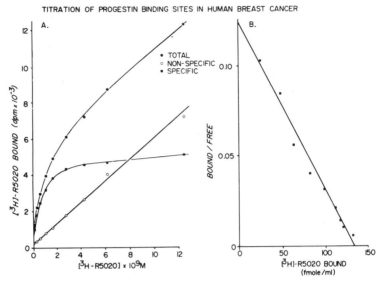

Fig. 1: Titration analysis of estrogen receptors in human breast carcinoma.
A. Aliquots (0.1 ml) of cytosol prepared from frozen human breast tumors were incubated in triplicate with 0.1 ml ^{3}H-R5020 solutions in homogenization buffer containing increasing amounts of radioactive ligand either in the absence (●) or presence (○) of a 200-fold excess of R5020. Specific binding (■) was estimated as the difference between total binding and binding in the presence of the competitor.
B. The titration data from A were plotted according to the method of Scatchard. The dissociation constant (K_d) determined from the slope of the curve was 1.1×10^{-9}M for this preparation. The binding capacity of the progestin receptor complexes was estimated from the intercept on the abscissa and gave a value of 74 fmol/mg cytosol protein.

estrogen binding capacities of > 10 fmol of estrogen bound appear to represent a "receptor positive" tumor.

The sucrose gradient method which separates the various forms of the steroid receptors assesses certain molecular properties of these proteins in a tumor extract (Fig. 2). Using this method, it has been determined that the sedimentation profiles of both estrogen and progestin receptors in human breast carcinomas fall into four general categories (Jensen *et al.*, 1971; Wittliff, 1974). These are tumors which contain specific steroid binding components migrating at either 8S, 4S or both 8S and 4S (Fig. 2) and those in which receptors are undetectable. A more accurate estimation of the sedimentation coefficients of these molecular forms has been made using a number of marker proteins (Wittliff, 1975 & 1978). From these data the higher molecular weight species of the estrogen receptor sedimented

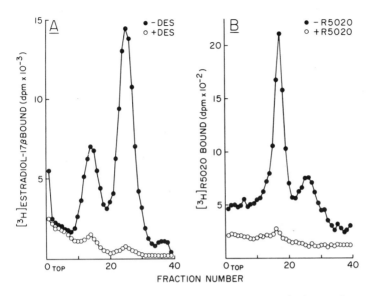

Fig. 2: Sucrose gradient separation of estrogen and progestin (R5020) receptors in human breast carcinoma.

Tumor cytosol was reacted either with ^{3}H-estradiol (A) or with ^{3}H-R5020 (B) for 4 hr at 3°C in the presence (○) or absence (●) of a 200-fold excess of unlabeled competitor. Note the presence of both 8S and 4S forms of these steroid receptors in the single breast carcinoma analyzed.

at 7.6-8.1S while the lower molecular weight form sedimented at 4.0-4.6S under conditions of low ionic strenght. Occasionally we have observed specific estrogen binding components sedimenting at < 4S (Wittliff *et al.*, 1978) under these same conditons. Some investigators have used the sucrose gradient method to quantitate the steroid binding capacity of human breast tumors (Jensen *et al.*, 1975; Wittliff *et al.*, 1972). When a saturating concentration of ^{3}H-ligand as well as an excess of a competitor used in this assay, the estimation of specific binding capacity is in good agreement with that determined by the titration analyses (Wittliff *et al.*, 1975).

Clinical utility

Data presented at the recent Consensus Development Conference on Steroid Receptors in Breast Cancer (Anonymous, 1979) clearly supported the findings from the earlier meeting in 1974 (McGuire, 1975) that breast cancer patients with tumors containing estrogen receptors were more likely to respond to endocrine manipulation than those whose tumor lacked these marker proteins. Since about 1975, determinations of estrogen receptors have been used along with certain clinical criteria such as menopausal status, site of the dominant metastatic lesions, response to previous hormone therapy and disease free interval in the management of breast carcinoma. More recently, as summarized at the Consensus Development Conference (1979) both the quantitative levels of estrogen receptors and the presence of progestin receptors in a tumor biopsy enhanced the accuracy of selecting a patient likely to respond to a hormonal therapy.

Currently both of these steroid receptors are being analyzed in thousands of breast tumor biopsies annually in the United States alone. As a means of examining the correlations of these data with responses to specific therapeutic modalities, certain clinical cooperative groups, particularly the National Surgical Adjuvant Breast Project (NSABP) and the Southeastern Cancer Study Group (SECSG) have initiated experimental therapeutic protocols requiring analyses of estrogen and progestin receptors of breast tumors. Thus, the establishment of assay uniformity and quality control is imperative to insure meaningful correlations between laboratory results and clinical response.

Sources of variability in analyses

An extensive problem has been the lack of uniformity in the methods of receptor analyses in the clinical laboratory and in the expression of specific steroid binding data. Some of the common sources of variability in steroid receptor analyses by clinical laboratories which we have observed in the past five years are:

1) range of steroid ligand concentrations
2) concentration and type of competitive inhibitor
3) incubation time and temperature
4) concentration of cytosol protein and type of assay selected
5) type and concentration of dextran-coated charcoal utilized

In addition there are a number of other parameters that may complicate steroid receptor analyses if not properly controlled. Among these are:

1) metabolism of the ligand
2) contribution of nonspecific (low affinity, high capacity) binding
3) ligand-receptor dissociation
4) ligand association with specific serum proteins such as sex steroid binding globulin and corticosteroid binding globulin
5) thermal lability both in the biopsy and cell-free
6) ionic strength lability
7) occupancy of binding sites by endogenous hormone

8) receptor "inhibiting" substances
9) proteolysis

To insure accurate quantification of the number of steroid binding sites in a biopsy using a titration procedure and dextran-coated charcoal to remove unbound steroid, it is necessary to use a broad range of tritium-labeled ligand concentrations. These must include a sufficient number of points below the saturation level so that an interpretable Scatchard plot is generated (e.g. Fig. 1). From our experience with laboratories participating in the cooperative clinical trials, a considerable number used too many saturating concentrations of either ³H-estradiol or ³H-R5020 so that the points were "grouped" near the abscissa of the Scatchard plot making it difficult to accurately estimate the dissociation constant.

Another common source of variation is the concentration and type of competitive inhibitor used to estimate the contribution of nonspecific (low affinity, high capacity) binding. It appears this is largely due to contamination of tumor biopsies by necrotic material and blood which may contain albumin and other proteins known to associate with steroid hormones such as sex steroid binding globulin and corticosteroid binding globulin. Diethylstilbestrol is a potent synthetic estrogen which does not bind to plasma proteins with high affinity. Thus, it is a very useful inhibitor to use in estrogen receptor analyses (Fig. 3) since it only associates with intracellular binding components. The dissociation constant (K_d) of the diethylstilbestrol-receptor complexes in cytosol from breast tumors is approximately 10^{-9} M which is one order of magnitude higher than that of estradiol-receptor complexes (Wittliff, 1978). Routinely we use a 200-fold excess of unlabeled diethylstilbestrol in a titration assay.

A similar quantity of unlabeled R5020, a synthetic progestin is utilized to estimate low affinity, high capacity binding (Fig.1). Since R5020 and certain glucocorticoids may associate with similar binding sites (Wittliff, 1977), it is advisable to also add an excess of unlabeled hydrocortisone to these reactions when glucocorticoid receptors are suspected in the specimen. The principle advantage of utilizing ³H-R5020 as a ligand for the progestin receptor is that it does not associate to any great extent with corticosteroid binding globulin known to bind progesterone, the natural progestin (Raynaud, 1977). Furthermore, it does not dissociate readily from the progestin receptor of mammary gland (Wittlif, 1977) as has been observed for progesterone nor is it metabolized under the conditions of most clinical assays (Raynaud, 1977).

If the sucrose gradient procedure (Fig. 2) is used to quantify steroid receptors, one must be sure to use a saturating concentration of the

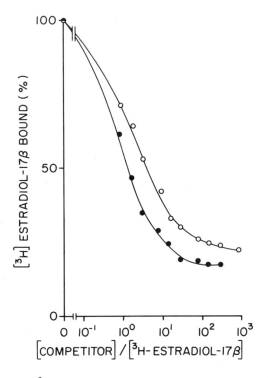

Fig. 3: Inhibition of ^{3}H-estradiol-17β binding in cytosol of human breast carcinoma by unlabeled competitors.

A constant volume of cytosol (0.1 ml) from human breast tumors was incubated in triplicate with 6.4 nmol/L ^{3}H-estradiol-17β either alone (●) in the presence of various concentrations of unlabeled estradiol-17β (●) or diethylstilbestrol (○). The steroids were dissolved in 0.1 ml homogenization buffer. Each point on the curves represents the mean of three determinations. The K_d calculated from a separate Scatchard analysis of titration data was 2.1×10^{-10}M. By means of the Rodbard relationship the estimated K_d of diethylstilbestrol-receptor complexes was 0.7×10^{-9}M.

tritium-labeled ligand, usually 3-5 nM for estradiol-17β or for R5020 as suggested from titration analyses (e.g., Fig. 1). Furthermore, it is imperative to use a competitive inhibitor of ligand binding to clearly estimate the receptor proteins. Since albumin and other contaminating proteins sediment in the 4S to 5S region of the sucrose gradient where certain receptor species migrate as well (e.g., Fig. 1 and Wittliff, 1977 & 1972), the ligand specificity should be evaluated.

To assess the estrogen specificity of the various molecular forms of the estrogen receptor, experiments were performed on the same cytosol preparation of human breast tumors using both ^{3}H-estradiol-

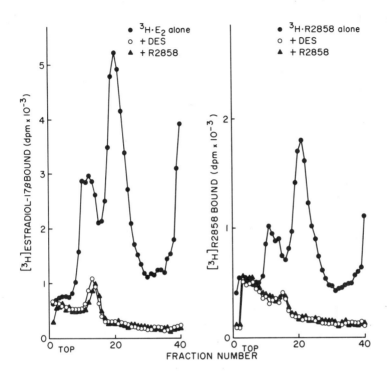

Fig. 4: Sucrose gradient centrifugation of estrogen receptors in human breast carcinoma.
The profiles in panel A represent cytosol incubated either with 5 nM ^{3}H-estradiol-17β alone (●) or in the presence of a 200-fold excess of unlabeled diethylstilbestrol (○) or unlabeled R2858 (▲) and separated on linear gradients of 10-35% (w/w) sucrose for 16 hr at 369,000 x g (3°C). Gradients described in panel B represent reactions incubated with 5 nM ^{3}H-R2858 alone (●) or in the presence of a 200-fold excess of diethylstilbestrol (○) or R2858 (▲). (Taken from Wittliff *et al.*, 1978).

-17β and a synthetic estrogen,^{3}H-R2858 (Raynaud, 1977). Using sucrose gradient centrifugation, the sedimentation profiles of estrogen receptors were examined using these two estrogenic ligands(Fig.4). Regardless of the ligand used, the estrogen receptor profiles were similar. Furthermore, both unlabeled diethylstilbestrol and R2858 inhibited either ^{3}H-estradiol or ^{3}H-R2858 binding to the same extent (Fig. 4).

As an additional criterion that these molecular components associate with estrogenic ligands with the same affinity and to the same extent, cytosols from human breast carcinomas were titrated with ^{3}H-estradiol using either unlabeled diethylstilbestrol or R2858 as inhibitors (Fig. 5). Separate experiments were conducted in which

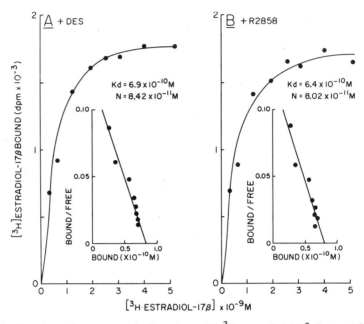

Fig. 5: Titration of estrogen binding sites with ^{3}H-estradiol-17β. Cytosol from a human breast carcinoma was incubated with increasing concentration of ^{3}H-estradiol-17β either alone or in the presence of an excess of unlabeled diethylstilbestrol (Panel A) or unlabeled R2858 (Panel B) for 16-18 hr at 3°C. Only specific binding data are presented. The insert in each panel describes the Scatchard plots of these specific binding data. K_d refers to the apparent dissociation constant while N represents the number of binding sites estimated from the intercept on the abscissa. (Taken from Wittliff *et al.*, 1978).

the same cytosol was titrated with ^{3}H-R2858 in the presence of either unlabeled diethylstilbestrol or R2858. Again, regardless of the estrogenic ligand used, when either diethylstilbestrol or R2858 was used as the inhibitor, similar affinities were observed (Fig. 5). Using ^{3}H-estradiol, the K_d was 6-7 x 10^{-10}M, and using ^{3}H-R2858 it was 7-9 x 10^{-9}M, indicating a difference in the affinities of these two ligands. However, similar specific binding capacities were observed when either ligand was used (Fig. 5). These data from the titration experiments and the sucrose gradient determinations (Fig. 4) suggest that both of the molecular forms of these receptors commonly observed on sucrose gradients may be considered specific estrogen binding entities.

In 1969 the principal author and his coworkers began a long term study to examine the original hypothesis set forth by Jensen and colleagues (Jensen *et al.*, 1971) that the presence of specific estrogen binding components in breast carcinomas was predictive of a patient's response to endocrine therapy. Using sucrose gradient separation of specific estrogen binding proteins in cytosol fractions of biopsies of primary and metastatic breast carcinomas, four types of receptor profiles have been demonstrated (Wittliff, 1974 & 1975). The majority of breast tumors containing estrogen receptors exhibited either the 8S species alone or both the 8S and 4S forms (Fig. 2). From 10-15% of breast carcinomas contained only the 4S type of estrogen receptor using sucrose gradients of low ionic strength (Wittliff *et al.*, 1976 & 1975). In spite of the differences in sedimentation properties, the ligand binding specificities and affinities of the 8S and 4S species of estrogen receptors were similar. The fourth category comprising approximately half of the infiltrating ductal carcinomas of the breast examined were those that did not contain any type of estrogen binding component.

Sherman *et al.* (1978) suggested these lower molecular weight forms represent proteolytic cleavage products of the other receptor species. If the distribution of the molecular species of steroid receptors is influenced by proteolytic activity in the cytosol, it may be ascertained by using a protease inhibitor. Antipain and leupeptin, peptides isolated from actinomycetes (Aoyagi *et al.*, 1969) appear to be useful for this purpose as well as aid in determining if proteolysis damages the ligand binding domain of the receptor. To determine if the 4S or the 4.5S components observed under low ionic strength conditions resulted from proteolytic cleavage of the 8S binding component, homogenates of a tumor powder were prepared either with 1mM leupeptin or in buffer alone. After separation of the cytosols by centrifugation, specific estrogen binding sites were associated with ^{3}H-estradiol and the unbound steroid removed with pellets of dextran-coated charcoal. Samples of the two reactions were separated on linear gradients of sucrose and the specific estrogen binding profiles were examined (Fig. 6). In addition to the 8S species, both 4S and 4.5S entities were identified under low salt conditions. In the presence of leupeptin, an increase was observed in the quantity of the 8S component. The extent of binding by the 4.5S component was not altered significantly, although the quantity of steroid bound by the 4S component was diminished considerably. In this experiment the total binding capacities of the two reactions were similar within 10%. Similar results were observed in other experiments conducted with identical conditions. Again, these data indicate that although proteolytic cleavage of the 8S estrogen receptor may occur under low ionic strength conditions, there is no change in the specific binding capacities. It appears that if the lower molecular weight

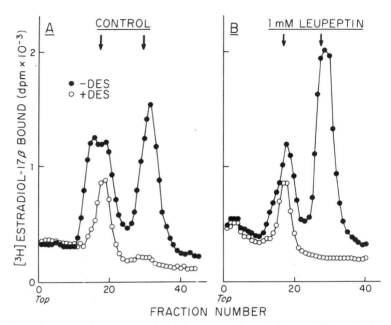

Fig. 6: Influence of a protease inhibitor on sedimentation profiles of estrogen receptors in human breast carcinomas. Using routine buffer conditions., homogenates were prepared either with 1 mM leupeptin (B) or without (A). Cytosols previously incubated either with 5 nM ³H-estradiol alone (●) or in the presence of 1 μM diethylstilbestrol (○) were separated on linear sucrose gradients by centrifugation for 16 hr at 3°C. The arrows indicate marker proteins sedimenting at 4.6S and 7.9S (Taken from Wittliff *et al.*, 1978).

forms of estrogen receptors are cleavage products, they retain the full capacity to associate with ³H-estradiol. Thus, routine addition of leupeptin to assay mixtures does not appear necessary nor financially practical for estimating steroid binding capacities.

A final but critical concern which often is a source of considerable variation in steroid receptor analyses is the selection and handling of breast tumor specimens. A number of years ago we developed protocols for these procedures which are in practice today. (Wittliff *et al.*, 1976, 1972 & 1975). Since human breast tumors are heterogeneous with regard to cell type, we examined the relationship between estrogen-binding capacity and the proportion of tumor epithelium in a breast biopsy (Fig. 7). From these data there does not appear to be a correlation between the quantity of estrogen receptors in a breast biopsy and the proportion of tumor epithelium. It was noted that numerous tumor specimens containing less than 25% tumor epithelium exhibited very high estrogen binding capacities.

RELATIONSHIP BETWEEN ESTROGEN-BINDING
CAPACITY AND PROPORTION OF TUMOR
EPITHELIUM IN BREAST TUMORS

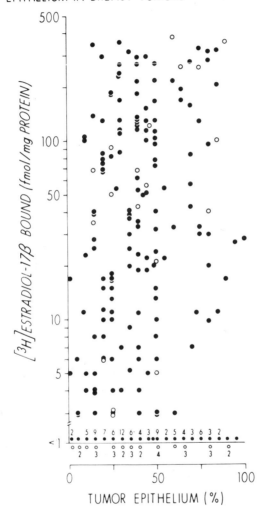

Fig. 7: Relationship between specific estrogen-binding capacity and proportion of tumor epithelium in human breast tumors.

At the time of estrogen receptor analysis, a representative sample of breast tumor was fixed in neutral formalin and processed for histologic examination. Relative concentration of tumor epithelium was estimated in specimens of primary (●) and metastatic (○) breast carcinoma and compared with estrogen-binding capacity. (Taken from Wittliff *et al.*, 1976).

Secondly, these data indicated that the specific estrogen-binding capacities of individual tumor specimens containing the same quantity of tumor epithelium were highly variable. As shown, the quantity of estrogen receptors in these tumors may vary from an undetectable level to one in excess of 100 fmol/mg cytosol protein. Although one may expect that the estrogen-binding capacity of normal mammary gland increases with increasing cellularity, this is not true of breast tumors. Thus, the quantitative differences in estrogen-binding capacity reported earlier (McGuire, 1975) were not due simply to the number of tumor cells in a biopsy. Rather, this variation in activity reflects differences in the number of binding sites per breast tumor cell.

The thermostability of steroid receptors in tumor biopsies has been difficult to assess, partially due to the heterogeneous nature of the tissue and the quantity of steroid receptors. However, it is clear from studies *in vitro* that steroid receptors are labile proteins which undergo degradation and/or ligand dissociation in a temperature dependent manner (Wittliff *et al.*, 1976). Association of the ligand with the receptor clearly aids in stabilization suggesting the time between cytosol preparation and introduction of the ligand should be as short as possible. Use of the vertical tube rotors for sucrose gradient centrifugation (Wittliff, 1977) and of the Beckman Airfuge for the preparation of cytosol (Heidemann *et al.*, 1979) eliminates most of this problem. Furthermore, the vertical tube rotor procedure (Wittliff, 1977) aids in reducing the dissociation of steroid-hormone receptor complexes likely to occur during overnight centrifugation of certain species.

Preparation, evaluation and distribution of tissue reference powders

Tissue reference powders composed of various quantities of frozen, pulverized organs such as uterus, breast, muscle and liver as well as certain types of sera (e.g., of pregnancy) were generated using several types of tissue grinders and liquid nitrogen. Breast tumors also were added to certain powders. Each of these reference powders was formulated in such a manner to contain different combinations of estrogen and progestin receptors, i.e., estrogen receptor positive, progestin receptor negative; estrogen receptor positive, progestin receptor positive, etc. Routinely, a laboratory from an institution participating in the cooperative trial of the NSABP or the SECSG is sent a set of two to four tissue powders frozen in dry ice. Often 4-5 vials of each powder are included to evaluate the assay variability of each receptor measurement. The laboratory analyzes these using "in house" methodology and returns the results to the headquarters of the NSABP or of the SECSG for comparison with data generated by other laboratories in the Cooperative Group and by the Reference Laboratory at the University of Louisville. Presently, either tolerance limits or confidence intervals are computed from the specific steroid binding capacities of each powder using titration analyses and dextran-coated charcoal. These data provide preliminary guidelines regarding the determination of agreement of assay results among the laboratories of the Cooperative Groups. Tolerance limits appear to more accurately express agreement in statistical terms but require considerably more analyses by both the Reference Laboratory and the participating clinical laboratory. The dextran-coated charcoal procedure appears to be the most widely utilized for estimating estrogen and progestin receptors of human breast tumors by clinical laboratories in the United States and Canada.

Furthermore, if a laboratory used by a member of the NSABP or of the SECSG needs assistance with the development of a receptor procedure or with the modification of an established method, our laboratory also accomodates them either at the University of Louisville or at their institution. Thus far, we have participated in the establishment of uniformity in steroid receptor analyses in more than one-hundred laboratories in North America and in the development of steroid receptor reference facilities at the University of Düsseldorf in West Germany and at the University of Insbruck Frauenklinik in Austria.

An important consideration every laboratory contributing data to a cooperative treatment trial must evaluate is the extent of variability expected in steroid receptor analyses. To determine the amount of variation we suggest that each person measuring steroid receptors in a clinical laboratory estimate the receptor content on a series of tissue reference powders using at least three titration analyses. The results of such an experiment whereby five different individuals performed three separate estrogen receptor analyses on three different tissue reference powders is shown in Table I. The random variation within the powders determined from the data in Table I was 30.4 fmol/mg cytosol protein for this particular experiment (Table II). Surprisingly, the amount of variation in the results estimated between the five individuals participating in this experiment was less than the amount of random variation expected, i.e. 10.7 fmol/mg cytosol protein. These types of data are useful in bringing about quality control within a laboratory. We recommend that each facility analyzing steroid receptors in clinical material develop a tissue reference powder for daily monitoring of procedures. Because of the lability of these intracellular proteins, the selection of a

TABLE I

Analyses of estrogen receptors in reference powders used to establish
uniformity of these assays in clinical trials

Technician	reference powder		
	no.1	no.2	no.3
no. 1	262 ± 15 [a]	189 ± 48	59 ± 6
no. 2	208 ± 11	149 ± 9	70 ± 9
no. 3	227 ± 18	138 ± 3	63 ± 5
no. 4	234 ± 18	181 ± 8	74 ± 5
no. 5	190 ± 31	153 ± 6	65 ± 3

[a]Mean ± standard error of three determinations expressed as fmol/mg cytosol
protein. Specific estrogen binding capacity was determined by multiple concentration titration analyses using the dextran-coated charcoal procedure. (Taken
from Wittliff *et al.*, 1980).

TABLE II

Sources of variation in the analyses of estrogen receptors in reference powders

Sources of variation	amount of variation
Between Technicians	10.7[a]
Within Powders (Random)	30.4

[a]Expressed as fmol/mg cytosol protein using the data given in Table 1.

tissue for prepartion of the reference powder is critical. We have had
good experience with calf uterus frozen in liquid nitrogen shortly
after removal and pulverized while in the frozen state. Several of our
internal quality control powders have remained stable for more than
three months at -86°C with regard to estrogen and progestin receptor
levels. As an example from one powder, the mean ± standard deviat-
ion of the specific estrogen binding capacity was 131 ± 21 fmol/mg
cytosol protein (Fig. 8) and that of the progestin binding capacity
was 572 ± 141 fmol/mg cytosol protein (Fig. 9) when analyzed
weekly for a period of 120 days. Also, we have evaluated the use of
lyophilized calf uterus. The advantage of a tissue powder over a reference cytosol or a lyophilyzed tissue is that it permits evaluation of
the homogenizing procedure, clearly a critical step in the quantification of steroid receptor analyses.

From the studies of a multitude of investigators as well as those of
the authors, both the quality (integrity) and quantity (number of
binding sites) of estrogen receptors appear to be important as predictive indices when the oncologist is faced with the selection of a

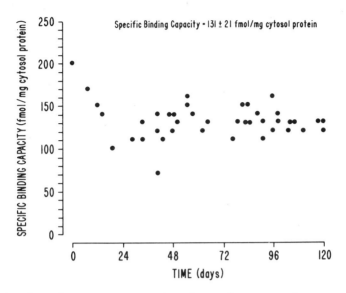

Fig. 8: Stability of estrogen receptors in a tissue reference powder.
At periodic intervals samples were analyzed for the quantity and affinity of estrogen receptors using a titration assay similar to that described in Fig. 1.

therapy likely to produce an objective remission. These latter considerations clearly impose a requirement for rigid quality control of steroid receptor analyses in the clinical laboratory.

Acknowledgements

The authors acknowledge the efforts of Dr. P. A. Wheeler-Feldhoff, Mr. D. T. Baker, Jr., Ms. L. N. Kane, Mr. M. L. Hall III, N. C. Clements, Jr. and J. B. Eckman, Jr. who have made important contributions to the Reference Powder Program. The valuable assistance of Mitzie Wittliff with organizational and secretarial aspects of the program is appreciated. Portions of these studies were supported in part by a developmental grant from the American Cancer Society and by funds from USPHS Grants CB-28376 and CA-19657 awarded by the National Cancer Institute.

References

Anonymous (1979). Consensus Development Conference Report, New Engl. *J. Med.* **301**, 1011-1012.
Aoyagi, T., Tekeuchi, T., Matsuzake, A., Kawamura, K., Kondo, S., Hamada, M., Maeda, K., and Umezawa, H. (1969). *J. Antibiot.* **22**, 283-286.
Heidemann, P., and Wittliff, J. L. (1979). *Clin. Chem.* **25**, 622-625.

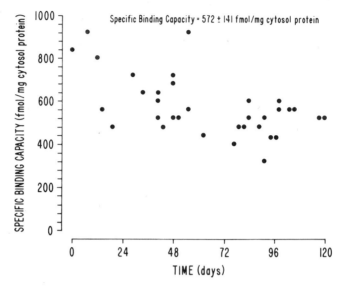

Fig. 9: Stability of progestin receptors in a tissue reference powder.
The quantity and affinity of ^{3}H-R5020 binding components were determined at periodic intervals using a titration assay similar to that described in Fig. 1.

Jensen, E. V., Block, G. E., Smith, S., Kyser, K., and DeSombre, E. R. (1971). *Natl. Cancer Inst. Monogr.* **34**, 55-79.

Jensen, E. V., Polley, T. Z., Smith, S., Block, G. E., Ferguson, D. J., and DeSombre, E. R. (1975). *In "Estrogen Receptors in Human Breast Cancer",* (W. L. McGuire, P. P. Carbone and E. P. Vollmer, eds.), p. 37-56. Raven Press, New York.

McGuire, W. L. (ed.) (1978). *In "Hormones, Receptors and Breast Cancer",* Raven Press, New York.

McGuire, W. L., Carbone, P. P., and Vollmer, E. P. (eds.) (1975). *Estrogen Receptors in Human Breast Cancer,* Raven Press, New York.

Raynaud, J. P. (1977). *In "Progesterone Receptors in Normal and Neoplastic Tissues",* (W. L. McGuire, J. P. Raynaud and E. E. Baulieu, eds.) p. 9-21. Raven Press, New York.

Sherman, M. R., Pickering, L. A., Rollwagen, F. M., and Miller, L. K. (1978). *Fed. Proc.* **37**, 167-173.

Wittliff, J. L. (1974). *Sem. Oncol.* **1**, 109-119.

Wittliff, J. L. (1975). *In "Methods in Cancer Research",* (H. Busch, ed.) Vol. XI, p. 298-354. Academic Press, New York.

Wittliff, J. L. (1977). *Applications Data,* Beckman Instruments, Inc. Spinco DS-509.

Wittliff, J. L., Beatty, B. W., Savlov, E. D., Patterson, W. B., and Cooper, R. A. Jr. (1976). *In "Recent Results in Cancer Research",* (G. St. Arneault, P. Band., and L. Israel, eds.), p. 59-77. Springer-Verlag.

Wittliff, J. L., Hilf, R., Brooks, W. F., Jr., Savlov, E. D., Hall, T. C., and Orlando, R. A. (1972). *Cancer Res.* **32**, 1983-1992.

Wittliff, J. L., Lewko, W. M., Park, D. C., Kute, T. E., Baker, D. T., Jr., and

Kane, L. N. (1978). *In "Hormones, Receptors and Breast Cancer"* (W. L. Mc Guire, ed.), Vol. **10**, p. 325-359. Raven Press, New York.

Wittliff, J. L., Mehta, R. G., Boyd, P. A., and Goral, J. E. (1976). *J. Toxicol. Environ, Hlth. Suppl.* **1**, 231-256.

Wittliff, J. L., Mehta, R. G., and Kute, T. E. (1977). *In "Progesterone Receptors in Normal and Neoplastic Tissues"* (W. L. McGuire, J. P. Raynaud, and E. E. Baulieu, eds.), p. 39-57. Raven Press, New York.

Wittliff, J. L., and Savlov, E. D. (1975). *In "Estrogen Receptors in Human Breast Cancer"* (W. L. McGuire, P. P. Carbone, and E. P. Vollmer, eds.), p. 73-91. Raven Press, New York.

Discussion

Janssen: Did you use progesterone or R5020 for the measurement of the progesterone receptor concentration?

Wittliff: We do the assays two ways. We use tritiated progesterone plus or minus unlabeled progesterone and to all of these mixtures we add hydrocortisone. More commonly we use tritiated R5020, plus or minus a 200 fold excess of R5020 with or without hydrocortisone. We tried various combinations in our assays, we occasionally even add androgens because of the properties R5020 has in some tissues. To answer your question we mostly use and recommend the tritiated R5020.

Griffiths: Do all the labs use the same methods and programs for the data handling?

Wittliff: The recommendation is that for the determination of the estrogen receptor a five point titration curve (five different concentrations) should be used plus or minus the inhibitor and the inhibitor used most often is diethylstilbestrol. For the progestin receptor a five point titration curve with R5020 plus or minus the inhibitor is recommended but there is no agreement on whether one should include hydrocortisone or not. We use a computer program with a linear regression curve for the nonspecific binding. We let the computer simply subtract this non-specific binding from the total binding and then plot these corrected values on a Scatchard plot.

Katzenellenbogen: Is there agreement on the data that people come up with in terms of affinity?

Wittliff: Maybe there is a small difference between the affinities of lyophilized tissues versus whole tissues that are frozen. But the agreement on the affinities is quite good and for the estrogen receptor these vary from 10^{-9} to as low as 10^{-11} M and for the progesterone receptor these are a little bit lower than that.

Katzenellenbogen: Is there a certain quantity of protein concentration under which these assays are run or do you let the labs choose there own?

Wittliff: We run all our assays at protein concentrations that are not lower than 2 and not higher than 5 but we prefer to stay around 3 to 4. The complication arises from the difference in the methods used to determine the protein concentration. Some people use the Lowry some use a biuret reaction. We use a microbiuret and this is the one that we find works best without any problems of sulphydryl-protecting reagents. You are right people may get the same number of absolute sites but when you measure the protein concentration in a different way you may get a different binding capacity per mg of protein.

Sandberg: What is the status of the nuclear receptor assay?

Wittliff: We have no quality control program that is set up formally for doing the nuclear ligand exchange procedure similar to the Anderson, Clark and Peck recommendation in the literature. We have a little quality control study going on in the lab in the lactating mammary gland. We prepare nuclei in glycerol and these are then frozen and with reasonable success we are able to use that as a quality control source for the nuclear ligand exchange procedure but only on the lactating mammary gland. We have tried to do this with human breast cancer but we haven't succeeded. I think the reason that we do not get the same kind of nuclei is that breast cancer is such a multivarious disease.

IN VITRO SCREENING FOR CYTOTOXIC ESTROGENS OF POTENTIAL THERAPEUTIC ACTIVITY

G. LECLERCQ, N. DEVLEESCHOUWER, N. LEGROS and J. C. HEUSON

Clinique et Laboratoire de Cancérologie Mammaire,
Service de Médecine,
Institut Jules Bordet, Brussels, Belgium

Introduction

We have recently initiated a screening programme for assessing the potential therapeutic value of new cytotoxic-linked estrogens for the treatment of breast cancer. This programme involves the following three points:

1. Drugs are first analysed *in vitro* for their binding ability to cytoplasmic estrogen-receptors (ER). Their stability in tissues (breast cancer, liver) and biological fluids are also examined. The biochemical assays used for that purpose (Leclercq *et al.,* 1976 & 1978) require only small amounts of drugs (1 - 10 mg) which need not be radioactively labeled. They are much simpler, cheaper and faster than classical pharmacological assays. They appear therefore especially appropriate for the screening of a large number of compounds.

2. When a drug is found to have both stability and significant binding affinity for ER, its specific cytostatic effectiveness is then investigated on the growth of two human breast cancer cell lines, one (MCF-7) containing ER, the other (Evsa-T) lacking ER (Lippman *et al.,* 1976). Only small amounts of drugs are again required for these *in vitro* studies.

3. The endocrinological properties and the toxicology of selected drugs are finally tested *in vivo* on mice and rats. Their potential antitumor effectiveness is also investigated on MXT-mouse mammary tumors and DMBA-induced rat mammary tumors. These two experimental systems are known to contain ER and be sensitive to hormone manipulations. Larger amounts of drugs are required ($\sim$ 5 g) to

conduct such experiments.

In previous studies (Leclercq *et al.*, 1976 & 1978) we reported that significant binding to ER occurred only with cytotoxic-linked estrogens having free oxygen functions in their estrogen moieties (hydroxyl groups for estradiol, diethylstilbestrol and hexestrol; hydroxyl and ketonic groups for estrone). Assuming that this property is an absolute requirement for a specific antitumor activity, we asked organic chemists to synthesize such compounds. So far 8 drugs have been produced (formulas on Table I).

The present paper is limited to the *in vitro* analysis of these 8 drugs. It reports and discusses their binding properties to ER. The potential antitumor activity of some of these is also investigated on the growth of MCF-7 and Evsa-T cells.

Material and methods

Compounds

Cytotoxic-linked estrogens were from the following origins: Ha compounds: Dr. H. Hamacher B. G. A., Berlin, Germany; E_1-Azi and E_2-bromoacetate: Dr. F. J. Zeelen, Organon Oss, The Netherlands; EC 10: Dr. R. Epzstein, Univ. Paris Sud, Orsay, France.

Estradiol-17β (E_2), estrone (E_1), hexestrol (HEX) and diethylstilbestrol (DES) were purchased from the Sigma Chemical Co.; Mustine-HCl from the Booths Co., Nottingham, U. K. Nafoxidine was supplied by the Upjohn Co, Kalamazoo, Mich.; Org 4333 by Organon, Oss, The Netherlands; $-N_3$ and $-NH_2$ derivatives of E_1 and HEX by Dr. G. Van Binst, V. U. B., Brussels, Belgium.

Cell lines

a) MCF-7*

Cytoplasmic and nuclear ER determinations confirmed the presence of receptors in MCF-7 cells (dextran-coated charcoal assay (E.O.R.T. C. 1973) and protamine assay (Chamness *et al.*, 1975). Cytoplasmic and nuclear ER concentration gave values close to those reported by other investigators (Horwitz *et al.*, 1978). Growth of the MCF-7 (see p. 169) was found to be only slightly stimulated by 10^{-8} M E_2 (0 to 20 %), the antiestrogen nafoxidine at 10^{-6} M and 5 x 10^{-7} M was always inhibitory (60 to 80 % and 40 to 60 % respectively). The inhibitory effect of nafoxidine was found to be reversed by 10^{-8} M E_2, E_1 and 11-chloromethylestradiol (ORG 4333), the latter estrogen being

---

* Supplied by Dr. M. Rich (Michigan Cancer Foundation, Detroit).

the strongest antagonist in this reaction (unpublished data).

b) Evsa-T

Evsa-T cells were supplied by Dr. M. E. Lippman (U S. National Cancer Institute, Bethesda, Md).

Cytoplasmic and nuclear ER determinations always failed to detect the presence of receptors. Growth of the cells were also found to be totally insensitive to E_2 and nafoxidine at concentrations ranging from 10^{-8} to 10^{-6} M.

Binding characteristics of the drugs

a) Apparent binding affinity

The apparent binding affinity of the drugs was measured by competitive inhibition of the binding of ^{3}H-E_2. These measures were performed with cytosol preparations from immature rat uterus. Parallel experiments with cytosol from DMBA-induced rat mammary tumors, human breast cancer or MCF-7 cells yielded similar results.

Since the experimental details of our assay have already been published (Leclercq *et al.*, 1976 & 1976), only the main steps will be given here. Cytosol was incubated at 18°C for 30 min. with 5 x 10^{-9} M ^{3}H-E_2 (saturating amounts) in absence or presence of increasing amounts of drug or unlabeled E_2 (control). After incubation, unbound compounds were removed by DCC and bound ^{3}H-E_2 was measured. The relative concentration of drug and unlabeled E_2 required to achieve 50% inhibition of the ^{3}H-E_2 binding gives its apparent binding affinity. In the case of a cytotoxic derivative of estrone (E_1), hexestrol (HEX) or diethylstilbestrol (DES), the parent estrogen was used as an additional control.

b) Reversibility of binding

Uterine cytosol was incubated overnight at 18°C with 5 x 10^{-9} M ^{3}H-E_2 in absence or presence of an excess of drug or unlabeled estrogen (control). After removal of unbound ligands by a DCC treatment, bound ^{3}H-E_2 was measured in an aliquot. Cytosol fractions were then again incubated at 18°C with ^{3}H-E_2 to allow ^{3}H-E_2 to exchange with reversibly bound ligands (Katzenellenbogen *et al.*, 1973). After 7 hours of incubation, which are sufficient for a significant exchange, cytosol fractions were treated with DCC and bound ^{3}H-E_2 was measured. Under these conditions, an increase in bound radioactivity in the exchange step indicates a reversible binding; an absence of increase in radioactivity indicates either an irreversible binding or a denaturation of the receptors.

TABLE I

Apparent binding affinity of compounds

	E_2 ($E_2 = 100$)	PARENT ESTROGEN (HEX, DES and $E_1 = 100$)
Ha IV	~ 0.01	~ 0.01
Ha V	~ 0.01	~ 0.01
Ha VI	0.5	3
Ha VII	0.5	3
E_2-Azi	3	
E_1-Azi	1	7
E_2-Bromoacetate	0.1	
EC 10	0.1	0.1

Effects of drugs on the growth of human breast cancer cell lines

MCF-7 and Evsa-T cells were grown in Falcon plastic flasks (75 sq cm) containing Earle's minimal essential medium (MEM) supplemented with 0.6 mg L-glutamine/ml, 40 μg gentamicin/ml, 100 U penicillin/ml, 100 μg streptomycin/ml and 10% fetal calf serum. At confluence, cells were removed by trypsinisation (trypsin 0.05%, EDTA 0.025%) and suspended (50 to 200,000 cell/ml) in the growth medium supplemented with charcoal stripped fetal calf serum (0.5% charcoal, 0.005% dextran in 1.5 ml medium/ml serum; overnight incubation at 4°C). Cells were then plated in 35 mm Petri dishes containing the same medium and cultured at 37°C in a humidified 95% air 5% CO_2 atmosphere. After 24 hours, drugs solubilised in ethanol were added to the culture dishes (final concentration of ethanol: 0.1%). Forty-eight hours later the medium was replaced by fresh drug-containing medium. The culture was then pursued for an additional 72 hour period before harvest. At that time, the cells were washed twice with 2 ml of Earle's base before being suspended in 1.5 ml trypsin-EDTA. Total DNA of collected cells was precipitated in 0.5N perchloric acid and evaluated by the diphenyl amine method (Burton, 1956). Cultures were run in quadruplicate for each experimental condition;

In brief, according to this protocol, the action of a drug on the growth of MCF-7 and Evsa-T cells was estimated by measuring the amounts of DNA after 120 hours of culture in presence of the drug. Cytotoxic-linked estrogens were used at concentrations of 10^{-8}M, 10^{-7} and 10^{-6}M. These concentrations were chosen because they cover the range in which E_2 and nafoxidine produce their effect in the MCF-7 cells.

Results

Binding characteristics of cytotoxic-linked estrogens

a) Apparent binding affinity

All cytotoxic-linked estrogens were found to be effective in the competitive inhibition test suggesting their binding to ER. Estimated apparent binding affinities are given in Table I.

Nitrogen mustard derivatives

The binitrogen mustard compounds Ha IV and Ha V were only found to produce a 50% reduction of ^{3}H-E_2 binding at a very high concentration ($> 10^{-5}$M). Exchange experiments indicated that these inhibitions were due to the compounds themselves and not to small amounts of contaminating parent estrogen (see below). Estimated apparent binding affinities were about 0.01% relative to E_2 and parent estrogens.

In contrast, the mononitrogen mustard compounds Ha VI and Ha VII produced a 50% reduction of ^{3}H-E$_2$ binding at concentrations of 10^{-6} to 10^{-5} M. Their apparent binding affinities were 3% relative to their parent estrogen (E_1).

Finally, in an additional control experiment, it was found that mustine-HCl failed to reduce ^{3}H-E$_2$ binding at concentrations as high as 10^{-3} M. This observation rules out the possibility that Ha compounds would simply act by a non-specific effect of their nitrogen mustard groups.

Aziridine derivatives

The two aziridine derivatives produced a 50% reduction of ^{3}H-E$_2$ binding at relatively low concentrations (E_2-Azi: 2 x 10^{-7} M; E_1-Azi. 7 x 10^{-7} M). Their estimated apparent binding affinity was about 5% of their parent estrogen.

Bromoacetate and epoxy derivatives

Both compounds produced a 50% reduction of ^{3}H-E$_2$ binding at concentrations close to 10^{-5} M indicating a low apparent binding affinity ($\sim 0.1\%$).

b) Stability of interaction of Ha compounds and E_1-Azi with estrogen receptors

The stability of drug binding to ER was studied in exchange experiments. Only Ha compounds and E_1-Azi have been submitted to this analysis (Fig. 1 - 3).

Fig. 1 and 2 show that Ha compounds and parent estrogens inhibited ^{3}H-E$_2$ binding in the first step of the experiment (black columns). As expected, this inhibition was less with Ha compounds than with parent estrogens in view of their lower apparent binding affinity. During the second phase of the experiment (open columns) there was a significant exchange of bound unlabeled estrogens by ^{3}H-E$_2$ indicating that their binding was reversible. This phenomenon did not occur with Ha compounds suggesting that they formed very stable complexes (apparently irreversible) with the receptors. Another explanation would be that these compounds denaturate the receptors so that they could no longer bind ^{3}H-E$_2$.

In contrast, under these experimental conditions, bound E_1-Azi was readily exchanged by ^{3}H-E$_2$ as its parent estrogen (Fig. 3). A totally

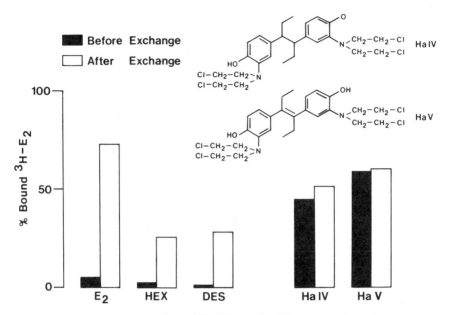

Fig. 1: Irreversibility of binding of Ha IV and Ha V compounds with cytoplasmic ER (Exchange experiment). Unlabeled E_2, DES and HEX (control of reversibility of binding) were at the concentration of 10^{-6}M; Ha IV and V at 10^{-4}M. On the graph, the activity is expressed in percent of bound ^{3}H-E_2 in absence of any unlabeled competitor.

reversible interaction must therefore be ascribed to this drug.

Effects of Ha compounds and E_1-Azi on MCF-7 and Evsa-T cell line.

The potential antitumor activity of Ha compounds and E_1-Azi on the growth of MCF-7 and Evsa-T breast cancer cell lines has already been examined. The activity of the other compounds, more recently received, is presently under investigation.

a) Ha compounds

At the concentration of 10^{-6} M, Ha compounds inhibited growth of the MCF-7 cells (Table II). The two bi-nitrogen mustard derivatives Ha IV and Ha V produced an inhibitory effect of about 35 to 40%; the mononitrogen mustard compounds Ha VI and Ha VII produced a stronger inhibition (about 80 to 90%). At lower concentrations, all drugs were devoid of significant effect except Ha VII which markedly inhibited growth at 10^{-7}M (45%). With regard to the Evsa-T cells, only Ha VII was found to inhibit growth ($\sim$ 80%) at 10^{-6} M indicating that these drugs had a weaker effect on this line than on the

TABLE II
Action of Ha compounds on growth of MCF-7 Evsa-T cells

DNA ($\mu g \pm S D$)

Molarity of drug	MCF-7				Evsa-T			
	Ha IV	Ha V	Ha VI	Ha VII	Ha IV	Ha V	Ha VI	Ha VII
NONE	10.4±1.4 (100)+	14.8±0.5 (100)	10.4±1.5 (100)	12.1±1.8 (100)	22.6±2.5 (100)	8.8±1.0 (100)	11.4±0.8 (100)	25.7±2.5 (100)
10^{-8}M	10.0±0.8 (96)	13.6±0.1 (92)	10.5±0.4 (101)	12.7±1.4 (105)	20.0±2.1 (88)	10.0±1.0 (114)	13.2±0.6 (116)	26.1±0.5 (102)
10^{-7}M	9.4±0.9 (90)	13.6±1.8 (92)	9.2±0.7 (88)	6.7±1.2 (55)	19.6±2.6 (87)	9.1±0.8 (103)	9.8±0.8 (86)	23.7±2.9 (92)
10^{-6}M	6.6±1.3 (64)	9.1±1.6 (62)	2.4±0.5 (23)	1.2±0.2 (10)	19.2±2.3 (85)	9.5±1.2 (108)	12.6±0.6 (110)	4.5±1.1 (18)

+ Per cent of control value

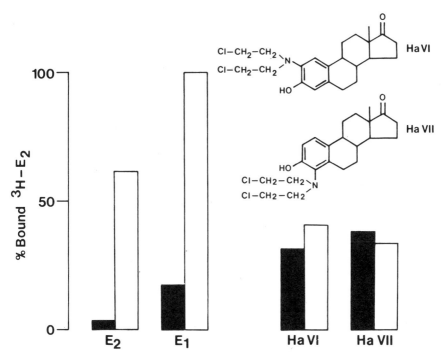

Fig. 2: Irreversibility of binding of Ha VI and Ha VII compounds with cytoplasmic ER (Exchange experiment). Unlabeled E_2 and E_1 (control of reversibility of binding) were at the concentration of 10^{-6}M; Ha VI and Ha VII at 10^{-5}M. On the graph, the activity is expressed in percent of bound ^{3}H-E_2 in absence of any unlabeled competitor.

MCF-7 one.

In contrast to Ha compounds, mustine-HCl was found to inhibit the growth of both MCF-7 and Evsa-T cells (Table III). This drug produced a significant effect at concentration about 1,000 times lower than Ha compounds indicating a higher cytotoxicity. Evsa-T cells appeared to be more sensitive than MCF-7 cells.

With regard to the MCF-7 cells, a series of E_1 and HEX derivatives linked with non-cytotoxic agents (-N_3, -NH_2) in the same position as the nitrogen mustard group were tested. All had a significant apparent binding affinity ($\sim$ 1-15% of their parent estrogen). None produced an inhibition of cell growth at the concentration of 10^{-6} M (Table IV).

Finally, in the MCF-7 cells, the possibility of a suppression by estrogens of the inhibitory effect of Ha compounds was analysed. E_2 and ORG 4333 were used for that purpose. The latter estrogen was

TABLE III
Inhibitory effect of mustine-HCl on MCF-7 and Evsa-T
Cell growth

Molarity of mustine	DNA ($\mu g \pm$ S.D.)	
	MCF-7	Evsa-T
NONE	5.7 ± 0.2 (100)+	8.6 ± 1.1 (100)+
10^{-13} M	4.7 ± 1.1 (82)	7.6 ± 0.9 (88)
10^{-11} M	3.0 ± 0.9 (53)	6.7 ± 0.8 (78)
10^{-9} M	3.5 ± 0.7 (61)	6.2 ± 1.0 (30)
10^{-7} M	3.1 ± 0.4 (54)	1.8 ± 1.2 (21)
10^{-6} M	3.8 ± 0.4 (67)	2.9 ± 0.3 (34)
10^{-5} M	-1.8 ± 0.3 (-32)	-2.2 ± 0.2 (-25)

+ Percent of control value.

TABLE IV
Comparison of non-cytotoxic analogues of Ha compounds
on growth of MCF-7 celles

Ha Compound	Analogue	DNA ($\mu g \pm$ S D)			
		Control	Ha Compound[++]	Control	Analogue[++]
Ha IV		10.4 ± 1.4	6.6 ± 1.3 (64)+	10.9 ± 1.0	11.4 ± 0.5 (104)
Ha VI		10.4 ± 1.5	2.4 ± 0.5 (23)	12.4 ± 0.8	14.1 ± 1.5 (114)
Ha VI		10.4 ± 1.5	2.4 ± 0.5 (23)	12.4 ± 0.8	12.0 ± 1.0 (97)
Ha VII		12.1 ± 1.8	1.2 ± 0.2 (10)	12.4 ± 0.8	11.7 ± 0.7 (94)
Ha VII		12.1 ± 1.8	1.2 ± 0.2 (10)	12.4 ± 0.8	12.0 ± 0.8 (97)

+ Percent of control value   ++ Concentration of the compounds: 10^{-6} M

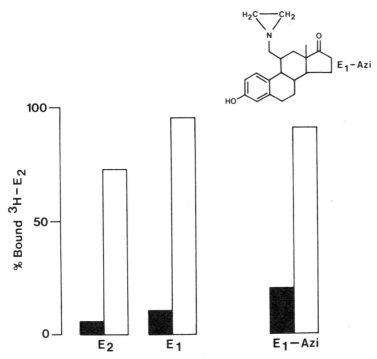

Fig. 3: Reversibility of binding of E_1-Azi with cytoplasmic ER (Exchange experiment). Unlabeled E_2 and E_1 (control of reversibility of binding) were at the concentration of 10^{-6}M; E_1-Azi at 10^{-5}M. On the graph the activity is expressed in percent of bound ^{3}H-E_2 in absence of any unlabeled competitor.

selected in view of its very high and stable interaction with ER (Fig. 4). A high antagonistic property towards the inhibition of nafoxidine on the MCF-7 cell growth also justified its use. Table V shows that E_2 as well as ORG 4333 at 10^{-8}M fail to reverse the inhibitory effect of 10^{-6}M Ha compounds.

b) E_1-Azi

The aziridine derivative E_1-Azi also influenced the growth of the MCF-7 cells. Concentrations of 10^{-8} and 10^{-7}M appeared stimulating ($\sim$ 40 and 30% respectively) whereas 10^{-6}M was slightly inhibitory (23%). With regard to the Evsa-T cells, no effect was observed at any concentration (Table VI).

Nafoxidine at 10^{-7}M was found to reverse the activating effect of the drug at 10^{-8}M; 10^{-8}M E_2 reversed its inhibiting effect at 10^{-6}M (Table VII).

TABLE V
Irreversibility of inhibitory effect of Ha compounds
on growth of MCF-7 cells

	Control	DNA (μg $\pm$ S D)		
		Ha Compound		
		alone	$+E_2$	$+ORG\ 4333^{++}$
Ha IV	12.3 ± 0.6	10.0 ± 0.2 (81)+	9.4 ± 0.6 (76)+	8.7 ± 1.6 (71)+
Ha V	12.3 ± 0.6	9.5 ± 1.0 (77)	8.8 ± 1.1 (72)	9.1 ± 0.8 (74)
Ha VI	12.9 ± 1.2	9.0 ± 0.3 (70)	6.8 ± 1.2 (53)	6.8 ± 0.9 (53)
Ha VII	17.2 ± 1.2	1.6 ± 0.3 (9)	1.6 ± 0.4 (9)	0.9 ± 0.5 (5)

+ Percent of control value
++Concentration of the compounds = Ha: 10^{-6}M; E_2 and ORG 4333: 10^{-8}M.

TABLE VI
Action of E_1-Azi on growth of MCF-7 and Evsa-T cells

	DNA (μg $\pm$ S D)	
Molarity of E_1-Azi	MCF - 7	Evsa-T
NONE	6.9 ± 1.0 (100)+	12.8 ± 0.8 (100)+
10^{-8}M	9.5 ± 0.5 (138)	12.8 ± 1.4 (100)
10^{-7}M	8.8 ± 1.3 (128)	13.6 ± 0.8 (106)
10^{-6}M	5.3 ± 1.0 (77)	12.0 ± 1.8 (94)

+ Percent of control value

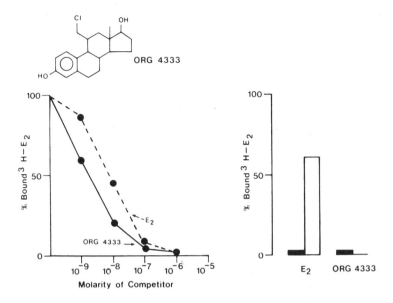

Fig. 4: Comparison of interaction of E_2 and ORG 4333 with cytoplasmic ER. Left: estimation of apparent binding affinity (competition between ^3H-E_2 and unlabeled E_2 and ORG 4333 for the binding to cytoplasmic ER). Right: reversibility of binding of E_2 and irreversibility of binding of ORG 4333 (Exchange experiment). On the graph, the activity is expressed in percent of bound ^3H-E_2 in absence of unlabeled E_2 and ORG 4333.

TABLE VII
Reversibility of effects of E_1-Azi on growth of MCF-7 cells

DNA ($\mu g \pm S\,D$)

Control $7.0 \pm 0.6\,(100)$

Stimulatory effect

E_1-Azi[++]
$9.8 \pm 0.6\,(140)$[+]

E_1-Azi + Nafoxidine[++]
$7.3 \pm 0.7\,(104)$

Inhibitory effect

E_1-Azi[++]
$5.2 \pm 0.8\,(74)$

E_1-Azi + E_2[++]
$6.8 \pm 0.9\,(97)$

+ Percent of control value
++ Concentration of the compounds:
   - stimulatory effect: E_1-Azi $10^{-8}M$, Nafoxidine $10^{-7}M$
   - inhibitory effect: E_1-Azi $10^{-6}M$, E_2 $10^{-8}M$

Discussion

The results reported here show that all drugs tested bind with ER. Estimation of their apparent binding affinity revealed a very large spectrum of values which cannot be easily explained on the basis of available data on the interaction of estrogens with ER (Geynet et al., 1972; Glusker, 1979). Our data, however, largely confirm the known fact that the chemical nature of a substituent largely influences the interaction of its parent estrogen with the receptors. This is demonstrated by the great difference in binding affinity between the aziridine and bromoacetate derivatives in which the substitution is in the same position (Katzenellenbogen, 1977) on the steroid. The position of the substitution also clearly influences the interaction of the estrogen with ER. In this regard, the large difference in affinity between the mono- and the binitrogen mustard derivatives highly suggests that significant interaction requires that at least one oxygen function of the estrogen moiety be free of any interaction with the cytotoxic agent. Finally, it seems likely that spatial configuration of the drugs plays an important role in their binding to the receptors. In flexible molecules such as HEX, important spatial modifications of the estrogen moiety may obviously occur from the linkage of the cytotoxic group. Such modications might be responsible for the unexpected low apparent binding affinity of EC 10.

Linkage of cytotoxic groups should also strongly modify the stability of the interaction of the estrogens with ER. In this regard, the high stability of the nitrogen mustard derivatives suggests an alkylation of the receptors by the cytotoxic agents. That chlorine atoms of the agent are involved in the reaction seems likely in view of the lack of a stable interaction with the aziridine derivative.

Assessment of the action of some of these drugs on the growth of the two breast cancer cell lines MCF-7 (ER+) and Evsa-T (ER−) revealed a marked inhibitory effect on the former line. These effects occurred at concentrations ranging from 10^{-8} to 10^{-6} M. These concentrations are exactly the same as those reported to produce effects in the MCF-7 cells in the case of estrogens and antiestrogens (Lippman et al., 1976; Zava et al., 1977; and our data). Both cell lines were also found to be very sensitive to the action of mustine-HCl. Concentration close to 10^{-9} M of the latter drug still produced a marked inhibitory effect especially in the Evsa-T line. All these data concur to suggest that tested cytotoxic-linked estrogens act mainly on growth as hormones rather than cytostatics.

With regard to the nitrogen mustard derivatives, it was found that the compounds having the highest apparent binding affinity for ER

(Ha VI and Ha VII) produced the strongest inhibition of the MCF-7 cells. This observation supports the hypothesis of a participation of ER in their cytotoxic action. That non-cytotoxic analogues did not inhibit the growth of the MCF-7 cells indicated that the nitrogen mustard of Ha compounds was directly involved in their cytotoxic action.

However, estradiol and ORG 4333 were unable to reverse the inhibitory effect of Ha compounds. This observation distinguishes the inhibitory effects of these drugs with those of a conventional antiestrogen (Lippman *et al.*, 1976) and, thereby, casts some doubt on the hypothesis of a participation of ER in this cytotoxic action. Indeed, a higher non specific cytotoxicity on the MCF-7 cell line cannot be excluded. On the other hand, the lack of sensitivity could also be explained by the very stable interaction of these drugs with ER which do not exist with conventional antiestrogens. Additional studies appear therefore needed to confirm the specific action of these drugs. Analysis of their effects on the growth of a variety of other cell lines either containing (i.e. ZR-75-1 (Engel *et al.*, 1978)) or lacking ER (i.e. G-11, MDA-231, MT-39 ... (Lippman *et al.* 1976)) should be the first step to solve the problem.

The aziridine derivative (E_1-Azi) either stimulated or slightly inhibited the growth of the MCF-7 cells depending upon the concentration used. It seems likely that ER mediated these effects since they were suppressed by nafoxidine and estradiol respectively.

In conclusion, all cytotoxic-linked estrogens tested in the present study bind to ER. Unfortunately, their large spectrum of apparent binding affinities hinders to draw major guide lines to be drawn for the synthesis of other drugs of very high affinity. With regard to the action of these cytotoxic-linked estrogens on the growth of human breast cancer cell lines, it seems that they display a stronger inhibitory effect on the estrogen sensitive cells suggesting that they may act through a mechanism involving ER. Additional studies are still needed to prove this hypothesis.

Acknowledgment

We wish to thank Drs. R. Epzstein, H. Hamacher, G. Van Binst and F. J. Zeelen for the gift of drugs.

This work was supported by a grant from the "Fonds Cancérologique de la Caisse Générale d'Epargne et de Retraite", Belgium and by the contract no 1-CM-53840 from the National Cancer Institute, Bethesda, Maryland.

References

Burton, K. (1956). *Biochem. J.* **62**, 315.
Chamness, G. C., Huff, K., and, McGuire, W. L. (1975). *Steroids* **25**, 627.
Engel, L. W., Young, N. A., Tralka, T. S., Lippman, M. E., O'Brien, S. J., and, Joyce, M. J. (1978). *Cancer Res.* **38**, 3352.
E.O.R.T.C. (1973). *Europ. J. Cancer* **9**, 379.
Geynet, C., Millet, C., Truong, H., and, Baulieu, E. E. (1972). *Gynec. Invest.* **3**, 2.
Glusker, J. P. (1979). In *"Biochemical Action of Hormones"* (G. Litwack, ed.). vol **6**, p. 122. Academic Press, New York.
Horwitz, K. B., Zava, D. T., Thilager, A. K., Jensen, E. M., and, McGuire, W. L. (1978). *Cancer Res.* **38**, 2434.
Katzenellenbogen, J. A., Johnson, H., J. Jr., and Carlson, K. E. (1973). *Biochemistry* **12**, 4092.
Katzenellenbogen, J. A., (1977). In *"Biochemical Action of Hormones"* (G. Litwack, ed.), vol. **4**, p. 2. Academic Press, New York.
Leclercq, G., Heuson, J. C., and Deboel, M. C. (1976). *Eur. J. Drug Metab. Pharmacokinet.* **1**, 77.
Leclercq, G., Deboel, M. C., and Heuson, J. C. (1976). *Int. J. Cancer* **18**, 750.
Leclercq, G., and Heuson, J. C. (1978). *Cancer Treat. Rep.* **62**, 1255.
Lippman, M. E., Bolan, G., and, Huff, K. (1976). *Cancer Res.* **36**, 4595.
Zava, D. T., Chamness, G. C., Horwitz, K. B., and, McGuire, W. L. (1977). **196**, 663.

Discussion

Wittliff: One real concern is that in all of the data you have presented us on the exchange reaction even with estradiol you got only a maximum of 70%.

Leclercq: Yes, that is a question of kinetics. I selected a time that gives a significant binding. I have not presented all the data.

Wittliff: At what temperature do you do the incubations?

Leclercq: 18°C for seven hours, but I have done experiments with longer incubation times.

Wittliff: How can you be sure that the compounds that you are testing don't have a different dissociation rate?

Leclercq. I don't have all the data here but what I want to show is that the compound is different from the classical estrogens (hyperbolic exchange curve). When we do the exchange experiments, these compounds don't exchange while the classical estrogens do, that is all we can say.

Katzenellenbogen: For how long did you preincubate your 11β-chloromethylestradiol?

Leclercq: There was no preincubation.

Catane: Could one explain the action of agents like Ha VII by the fact that it destroys the receptor?

Leclercq: That is a possibility.

Katzenellenbogen: In your cell culture experiments do high concentrations of estradiol inhibit the cell growth?

Leclercq: At the concentration used they don't. The inhibitory effect of estrogens mainly starts around 10^{-5} M and we stopped at 10^{-6} M. At these concentrations we didn't observe an inhibitory effect.

Könyves: Have you studied these compounds on *in vivo* models like the DMBA-induced tumors?

Leclercq: Presently not. We are planning to study this but we need larger amounts of the drugs to do *in vivo* testing. Generally we get only 10-20 mg and that is not enough. We need 1 or 2 grams of the compound.

BIOCHEMICAL EFFECTS OF CYTOTOXIC ESTROGENS AND CYTOTOXIC ANTIESTROGENS

K.GRIFFITHS, P. DAVIES, M. E. HARPER & R. I. NICHOLSON

Tenovus Institute for Cancer Research,
Welsh National School of Medicine,
Cardiff, U.K.

Introduction

Although it has long been recognised (Hunter, 1786) that the growth and function of the prostate gland is dependent upon the secretion of testosterone by the testis, it was only a few decades ago, following the experimental work of Huggins and his colleagues (Huggins, *et al.,* 1940; Huggins *et al.,* 1941 and Huggins *et al.,* 1941) that antiandrogen therapy in the form of orchidectomy or estrogen administration was introduced for the treatment of carcinoma of the prostate. It was recognised that malignant prostatic growth can be dependent upon androgen stimulation and the administration of diethylstilbestrol has been a conventional form of treatment for the management of the disease.

The precise mechanism by which diethylstilbestrol controls prostatic growth is not yet completely established but it is generally accepted that the major antiandrogenic effect is exercised indirectly *via* the pituitary (Griffiths *et al.,* 1979), suppressing LH secretion and thus decreasing the synthesis of testosterone by the testis. There is also evidence that at least part of the antiandrogenic effect of diethylstilbestrol results from a direct action on the testis (Oshima *et al.,* 1967; Danutra *et al.,* 1973 and Shimazaki *et al.,* 1965). Evidence that the estrogen directly influences prostatic tissue is more equivocal although there are studies (Danutra *et al.,* 1973; Danutra *et al,* 1973; Shimazaki *et al.,* 1965; Farnsworth 1969 and Leav *et al.,* 1971) that administration of estrogens markedly alters C_{19}-steroid metabolism by the prostate. It is generally believed that after administration of large doses of diethylstilbestrol diphosphate (Honvan), the free and active form of the hormone is released at the appropriate site within the prostatic cells by the phosphatases present in high. concentration, although to date, there is little evidence of such a concentration of the estrogen within the tissue. Experimental work from this laboratory has not been able to demonstrate an effect of diethylstilbestrol on the selective transfer of 5α-dihydrotestosterone to the nucleus of the prostate cell by the androgen receptor protein, although certain experiments have clearly indicated that after administration of [^{3}H]- diethylstilbestrol to men with prostatic carcinoma, the radiolabeled material could be extracted from the nuclei of the removed prostatic tissue.

It is however well established that certain compounds are able to decrease the specific uptake of estradiol-17β by mammary tumor tissue. These anti-estrogens, particularly tamoxifen, the trans isomer of 1-[p-(β-dimethylaminoethoxy)phenyl]-1,2-diphenylbut-1-ene,I.C.I. 46474, influence the selective translocation of estradiol by specific receptor protein molecules to the chromatin of the nucleus and thereby have a valuable role in the treatment of women with advanced carcinoma of the breast. Extensive studies by these laboratories (Nicholson *et al.*, 1980, 1976, 1977, 1977, 1978 & 1979) have provided an insight into the biochemical mechanisms by which tamoxifen exerts its effect. It was evident from the work that tamoxifen was effective in inhibiting the growth of the DMBA-induced rat mammary tumor (Fig. 1), that the tamoxifen was responsible for the translocation of estradiol-17β receptor to the nucleus (Nicholson *et al.*, 1976 & 1977) (Fig. 2) and over a short period of time, stimulated RNA synthesis (Nicholson *et al.*, 1977) resulting from transcription of the DNA template by RNA polymerases. From the investigations with DMBA-induced rat mammary tumors, it has been shown that increases in RNA polymerase II (synthesising DNA-like RNA) activity from tamoxifen administration are qualitatively similar to those produced after estradiol stimulation during the early increase in RNA synthesis. This transient rise in activity is obligatory for the subsequent elevation of RNA polymerase I (synthesising ribosomal rRNA) and then a major prolonged enhancement of RNA polymerase II (Borthwick *et al.*, 1975). Similar effects to those produced after estradiol stimulation are seen during the early phase of the second peak of activity although tamoxifen then appears unable to maintain this secondary stimulated rise (Nicholson *et al.*, 1977).

The results established however, the initial influx of the antiestrogen

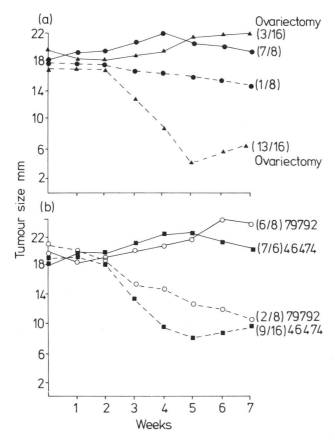

Fig. 1: The effect of ovariectomy and antioestrogens on DMBA-induced mammary tumor growth. Tumor size was measured weekly. Figs. in parentheses show the fraction of the tumors within a group that were either "growing" (———) or "regressing" (- - - - -); (a) ▲, ovariectomised; ●, sham operated. (b) Animals were injected daily for 14 days and then every 2 days for 5 weeks with 100 μg (per injection) of either I.C.I. 46,474 (■) or I.C.I. 79792 (o).

receptor complex into the nucleus and its relationship to transcriptional events. The possibility that such compounds as tamoxifen which may be selectively taken up by hormoneresponsive tumors, could be modified to carry into the nucleus a nitrogen mustard-containing grouping and localise a high concentration of this cytotoxic agent adjacent to the chromatin was considered in the early 1970's and two compounds, I.C.I. 85,966, (3,4-bis-(p-[(N-bis-2-chloroethyl) carbamoyl]-phenyl)hex-3-ene) and I.C.I. 79792, (1-(4-[β-bis-(2-chloroethyl)amino]ethoxyphenyl)-trans-diphenylbut-1-enehydrochlo-

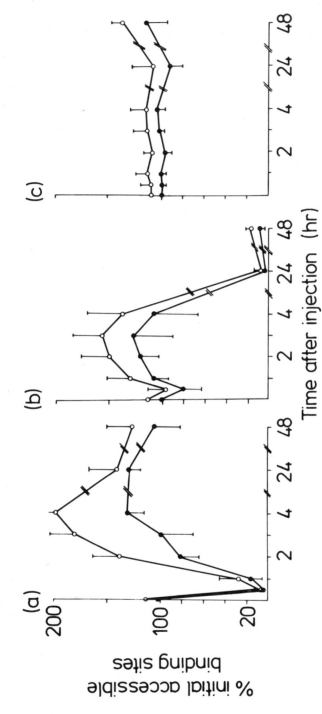

Fig. 2: Effect of *in vivo* administration of estradiol-17β and tamoxifen on the cytoplasmic levels of total and accesible estradiol-17β-binding sites. Rats were injected with either (a) 5 μg estradiol-17β (b) 100 μg tamoxifen (c) vehicle alone. Tumor biopsies were removed at the points indicated. Cytosol preparations from biopsies were incubated at either 4°C (accessible sites) (●) or 15°C (total sites) (○) for 120 mins with a saturating concentration of [³H] estradiol-17β (5.0 nmol/l) or [³H]- estradiol-17β plus 1000 fold excess unlabeled estradiol-17β. Results are expressed as a % of the value obtained by incubation of cytosol with labeled steroid at 4°C (accessible binding sites at time o) and is the mean ± SEM of 5 separate tumors.

ride) were made available to the laboratory by Dr. D. N. Richardson, I.C.I. Pharmaceuticals Ltd., Alderley Park, Cheshire. In Fig. 3 therefore are shown the structures of the nitrogen mustard-containing diethylstilbestrol and tamoxifen compounds and the following sections deal with certain aspects of their biochemistry.

Antiestrogens - effects in relation to rat mammary tumors

Mammary tumors were induced in virgin female Sprague-Dawley rats by intubation of DMBA (20 mg in 1.0 ml sesame oil). Approximately 7-12 weeks after intubation, tumors suitable for experimental purposes, (2 x 2 cm) were available. Minced tumors tissue (1 g) was incubated for 15 mins in Eagle's basal medium (10 ml/g) at 30°C in the presence of $[2,4,6,7^{-3}H]$-estradiol-17β (0.5 nmol/l, sp. act. 85 Ci/mmol) and with or without the addition of the non-radioactive antiestrogen or competitor (50 or 500 nmol/l). After incubation, the minced tissue was homogenised and nuclear pellets prepared

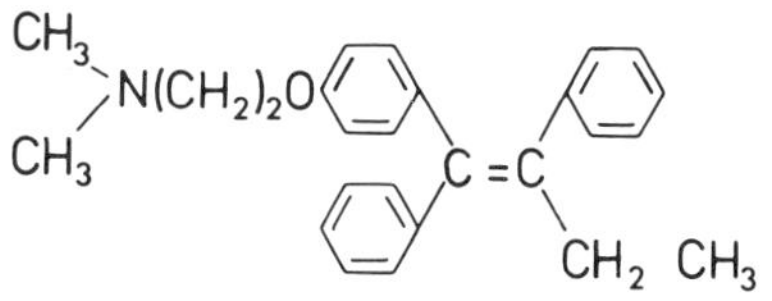

Tamoxifen (ICI 46474)

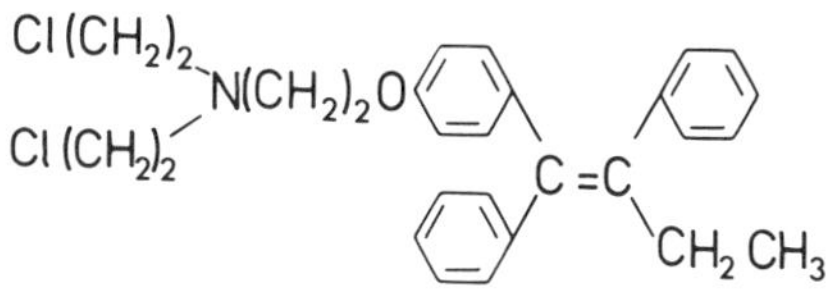

ICI 79792

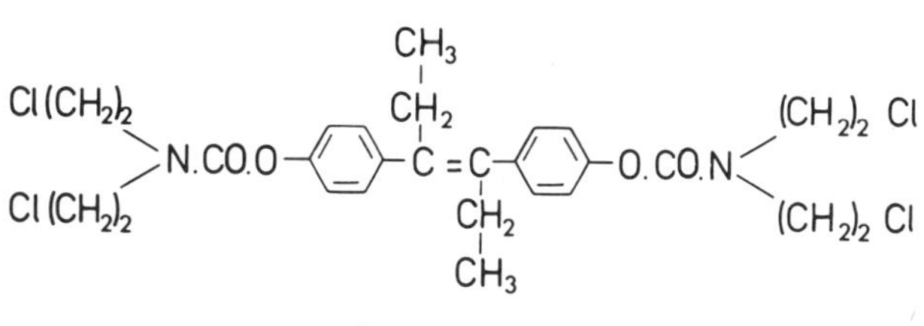

ICI 85966

Fig. 3: Structures of the various antiestrogens.

(Powell-Jones *et al.*, 1975). The nuclear preparation was extracted with 0.6 ml KCl (0.4 mol/l) at 4°C for 30 mins and aliquots of the extract analysed by sucrose density gradient centrifugation (Davies *et al.*, 1973).

After incubation of minced mammary tumor tissue with [³H] estradiol alone, a labeled steroid-receptor complex, sedimentation

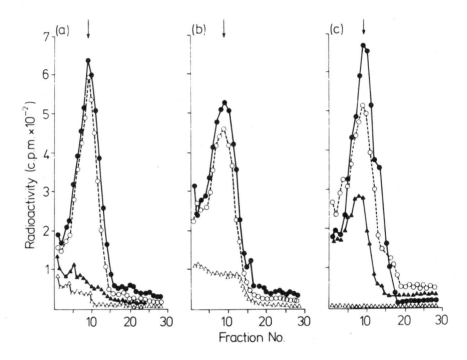

Fig. 4: Nuclear uptake of [³H]estradiol. (a) Mince incubated with [³H]estradiol alone (●) or with 50 nmol/l concentrations of unlabeled estradiol (△), diethylstilbestrol or dibutyldihydrostilbestrol (▲), or I.C.I. 46474, I.C.I. 79792 or I.C.I. 85966 (o). (b) Mince incubated with [³H]-estradiol alone (●), or with 50 nmol/l concentrations of unlabeled estradiol (△), or 500 nmol/l concentrations of I.C.I. 46474, I.C.I. 79792 or I.C.I. 85966 (o). (c) Mince preincubated (30 min at 30°C) with no additional substance (●), unlabeled estradiol (50 nmol/l (△), I.C.I. 46474 or I.C.I. 79792 (500 nmol/l) (o) or I.C.I. 85966 (500 nmol/l) (▲) before incubation with [³H]estradiol. Sedimentation marker (arrows) was in all cases bovine serum albumin ($S_{20,w}4.6S$).

coefficient 4-5S could be extracted (Fig. 4a). Although incubation in the presence of non-radioactive estradiol, diethylstilbestrol or another stilbestrol analogue, dihydrodibutylstilbestrol (50 nmol/l) inhibited this characteristic binding of [³H]estradiol, neither tamoxifen, I.C.I. 79792, nor I.C.I. 85966 at 50 or 500 nmol/l could produce a similar effect (Fig. 4; a and b). When minced mammary tumor tissue was pre-incubated with non-labeled competitor for 30 mins at 30°C before incubation with [³H]estradiol, tamoxifen, I.C.I. 79792 and I.C.I. 85966 inhibited the uptake of [³H]estradiol, the latter being the most effective (Fig. 4c).

These results are of interest in relation to further studies on the effect of these various compounds on the specific binding *in vitro* at 0°C, of [³H]estradiol (0.5 nM) by soluble supernatant cytosols prepared by centrifugation of rat mammary tumor homogenates at 100,000 g for 60 mins (Powell-Jones *et al.,* 1975).

Sucrose density gradient analysis of such [³H]estradiol-labeled cytosol preparations showed two peaks of protein-bound radio-activity corresponding to [³H]estradiol-receptor complexes of sedimentation coefficients 4S and 8S approximately (Fig. 5a) In-cubation in the presence of 100-fold excess non-radioactive estra-diol displaced the radioactivity of the specific 8S peak to the high-capacity 4S peak. A 100-fold excess (50 nM) of either diethylstil-bestrol or dihydrodibutylstilbestrol produced a similar effect (Fig. 5b). However, whereas 100-fold excess tamoxifen and I.C.I. 79792 effectively inhibited the binding of [³H]estradiol to its receptor at a 50 nM concentration (Fig. 6a), I.C.I. 85966 had no such ef-fect (Fig. 5a). Furthermore a 10-fold excess (5 nM) of diethyl-stilbestrol (Fig. 6b) and tamoxifen (Fig. 6c) also reduced the 8S-binding peak, whereas a similar concentration of I.C.I. 79792 had no effect (Fig. 6c).

The results would suggest therefore that since I.C.I. 85966 did not inhibit the specific binding of [³H]estradiol to these cytosols, the effect of the compound on the nuclear uptake of labeled es-trogen by whole-cell preparations probably reflects some degree of metabolism to diethylstilbestrol. In contrast, the ineffective-ness of tamoxifen and I.C.I. 79792 under these conditions in which whole-cell preparations were used may well be caused by their slower uptake by the cells compared to diethylstilbestrol, since both were effective in displacing estradiol from cytoplasmic re-ceptor protein, tamoxifen administration *in vivo* has been shown to decrease binding of [³H]estradiol by rat mammary tumor tis-sue (Nicholson *et al.,* 1975) and both inhibit the growth of these DMBA-induced tumors when administered *in vivo* (Fig. 1). Pos-sibly higher doses of I.C.I. 79792 could produce even more effec-tive inhibition of growth and further such studies may well be rewarding.

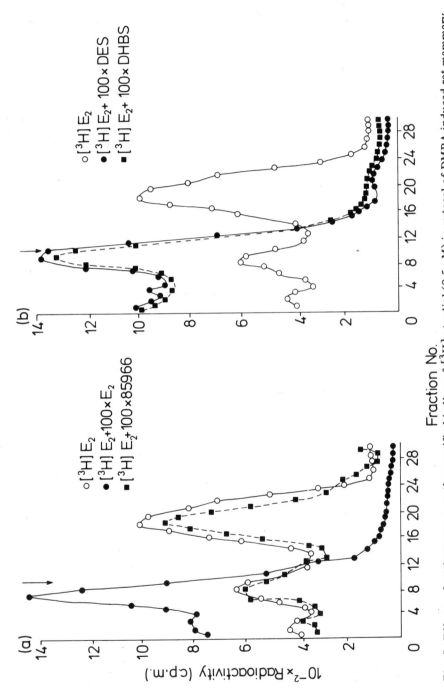

Fig. 5: Effects of antiestrogens on the specific binding of [³H]estradiol (0.5 nM) in cytosol of DMBA-induced rat mammary tumors. Sucrose density gradient centrifugation from left to right. The sedimentation marker was BSA ($S_{20,w}$ 4.6S).

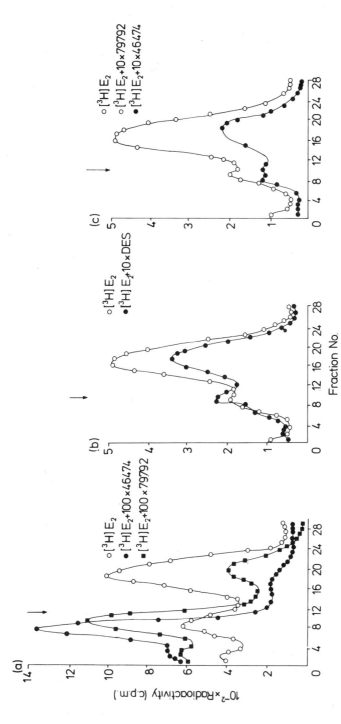

Fig. 6: Effects of antiestrogens on the specific binding of [³H]estradiol (0.5 nM) in cytosol of DMBA-induced rat mammary tumor. Sucrose density gradient centrifugation from left to right. The sedimentation marker was BSA ($S_{20,w}$4.6 **S**).

Androgens as possible carriers of cytotoxic agents

Androgenic steroids have been used in the treatment of advanced breast cancer and there are various reports relating to this (Jones, 1979; Hayward, 1970). The effects of androgens on rat mammary tumor growth has also been considered (Teller et al., 1968). In relation to this, early studies at the Institute and in other centres clearly established the paraendocrine behavior of human breast cancer and the capacity of such tissue to metabolise steroids. In particular, the studies in these laboratories showed the conversation of the adrenal secretory product dehydroepiandrosterone sulphate to various metabolites including androstene-5-ene-3β,-17β-diol and the 5α-androstanediols, of interest, since it has subsequently been shown that such C_{19} steroids competed effectively with [^{3}H]estradiol-17β for the cytoplasmic estradiol receptor protein isolated from DMBA-induced mammary tumors (Fig. 7) (Nicholson et al., 1978; Poortman et al., 1975). Furthermore, it was also shown (Nicholson et al., 1978) that androst-5-ene-3β, 17β-diol facilitated the nuclear translocation of the estrogen receptor although the transferred complex was found to have a relatively short nuclear retention time (Fig. 8). Later investigations in the Institute in which the C_{19} - steroid concentration of a series of human breast cancers was determined by high resolution gas chromatography-mass spectrometry (Maynard et al., 1976) indicated relatively high levels of both dehydroepi-androsterone and the androstenediol in certain of the tumors.

The possibility therefore exists to exploit the ability of the estradiol- 17β receptor protein to transfer certain C_{19}-steroid-nitrogen mustard derivatives to the nucleus of human breast cancer cells.

Cytotoxic estrogens and the prostate gland

Preliminary investigations at the Institute on the possible biochemical role of diethylstilbestrol and certain of its analogues suggested a possible inhibitory effect of such compounds on DNA nucleotidyltransferase (DNA polymerase) (Fahmy et al., 1968; Harper et al., 1970 & 1970). Similar studies established to investigate the biochemical effect of the androgen-receptor complex on isolated prostatic DNA-dependent RNA nucleotidyltransferase (RNA polymerase) (Davies et al., 1973 & 1972) indicated that the stilbestrol analogues also influenced the activity of the enzyme system (Davies et al., 1973) (Table I), and that I.C.I. 85,966 was equally as effective an inhibitor as diethylstilbestrol.

TABLE I

RNA Polymerase Activity (% change in activity)

Compound Added	Prostatic Nuclear Preparation		
Stimulation	Rat	Dog	Human
Testosterone	4	5	7
5α - DHT	43	21	42
5α - A - 3α17α - Diol	0	6	0
5αA-3α17β - Diol	33	0	2
5αA-3β,17α - Diol	0	0	0
5αA-3β,17β - Diol	35	2	32
Inhibitors			
Diethylstilbestrol	37	37	29
Estradiol	31	32	14
(±) - DHBS	-	-	0
Meso-DHBS	23	26	32
ICI-85966	-	-	30

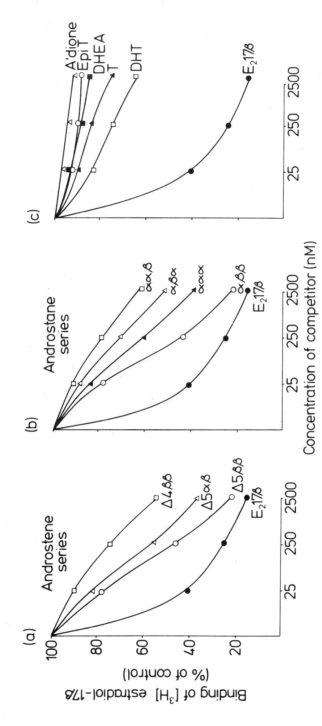

Fig. 7: Effects of various C_{19}-steroids on the binding of $[^3H]$estradiol in cytosol of DMBA-induced rat mammary tumors. $E_217\beta$ - estradiol: $\triangle 4\,\beta\,\beta$,androst- 4- ene-3$\beta$,17$\beta$ - diol: $\triangle 5\alpha\beta$, androst-5-ene-3α, 3β - diol: $\triangle 5\,\beta\,\beta$,androst-5-ene-3$\beta$,17$\beta$- diol: $\alpha\,\alpha\,\beta$, 5α - androstane-3α,17β - diol: $\alpha\,\beta\,\alpha$, 5α - androstane-3β, 17α - diol: $\alpha\,\alpha\,\alpha$, 5α - androstane-3α,17α- diol: $\alpha\,\beta\,\beta$, 5α androstane -3β, 17β - diol: A-dione, androstenedione; Epi-T, epitestosterone; DHEA, dehydroepiandrosterone: T, testosterone: DHT, 5α - dihydrotestosterone.

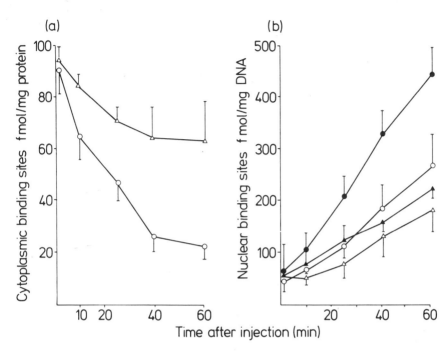

Fig. 8: Effect of *in vivo* administration of androst-5-ene-3β,17β - diol on cytoplasmic and nuclear estradiol-17β binding sites. Rats were injected with 100 μg (△) or 1 mg (○) at time 0 and tumor biopsy samples removed at varying time intervals thereafter. (a) Cytosol preparations from biopsies were incubated at 4°C for 16 h with a saturating concentration of [³H]estradiol-17β (5 nM) or [³H]estradiol-17β plus 1000-fold excess of diethylstilbestrol. (b) Nuclear fractions were incubated for either 4 hours at 15°C (●, ▲) or 16 hours at 4°C (○, △) with saturating concentrations of [³H]estradiol-17β (20 nM), with or without 1000 fold excess of diethylstilbestrol.

Extensive studies over a number of years have failed to indicate that diethylstilbestrol has any effect on the 5α-dihydrotestosterone-receptor interaction in prostatic tissue, although it does affect the metabolism of testosterone (Danutra *et al.*, 1973 & 1973), and it is still not yet evident that diethylstibestrol can be selectively taken up by prostatic tissue. There is evidence of an estrogen receptor in prostatic tissue (Wagner *et al.*, 1975; Hawkins *et al.*, 1975) but recent studies from the Institute (Chaisiri *et al.*) indicate that this may be localised in stromal tissue and not with epithelial cells.

Whether diethylstilbestrol plays any specific biochemical role in the prostatic cancer cell, which would influence tumor growth still requires elucidation and therefore the potential of such compounds as I.C.I. 85966 is uncertain. Administration of these compounds to rats showed that they influenced androgen-dependent tissues (Figs. 9 and 10) and plasma hormone levels (Fig. 11), but whether the effect of I.C.I. 85966 relates to its metabolism to diethylstilbestrol and its consequent inhibiting action in the pituitary is unclear. Further mass spectrometric analysis of prostatic tissue from animals given I.C.I. 85,966 would seem reasonable. Certainly hydrolysis of the estradiol-nitrogen mustard derivative Estracyt occurs after

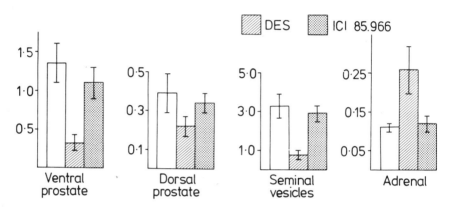

Fig. 9: Effect of diethylstilbestrol and I.C.I. 85,966 (100 μg/day for 10 days) on organ weights (mg/g initial body weight). Differences for diethylstilbestrol were significant (p < 0.005).

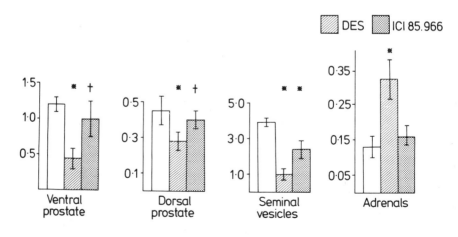

Fig. 10: Effect of diethylstilbestrol and I.C.I. 85,966 (500 μg/day for 10 days) on organ weights (mg/g initial body weight). Differences for diethylstilbestrol were significant (*p < 0.005 : + p < 0.050).

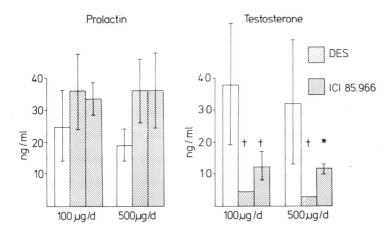

Fig. 11: Effect of diethylstilbestrol and I.C.I. 85,966 (100 μg/day for 10 days) on plasma prolactin and testosterone. ($+$ p $<$ 0.005; *p $<$ 0.050).

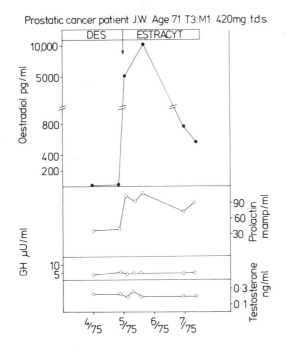

Fig. 12: Effect of Estracyt administration (420 mg t.d.s.) to a patient with prostatic cancer on plasma hormone levels.

administration to men with prostatic cancer (Fig. 12) and the analysis of intracellular components of the tumor tissue could offer increasing and valuable data.

Acknowledgements

The authors are grateful to the Tenovus Organisation for their generous financial support.

References

Borthwick, N. M. and Smellie, R. M. S., (1975). *Biochem. J.* **147**, 91.
Chaisiri, N., Valotaire, Y., Evans, B. A. J. and Pierrepoint, C. G. (Submitted for publication).
Danutra, V., Harper, M. E., Boyns, A. R., Cole, E. N., Brownsey, B. G. and Griffiths, K. (1973) *J. Endocr.* **57**, 207.
Danutra, V., Harper, M. E. and Griffiths, K. (1973). *J. Endocr.* **59**, 539.
Davies, P. and Griffiths, K. (1973). *Biochem. J.* **136**, 611.
Davies, P., Fahmy, A. R., Pierrepoint, C. G. and Griffiths, K. (1972). *Biochem. J.* **129**, 1167.
Davies, P. and Griffiths, K. (1973). *J. Endocrin.* **59**, 367.
Fahmy, A. R. and Griffiths, K. (1968). *Biochem. J.* **108**, 749.
Farnsworth, W. E. (1969). *Invest. Urol.* **6**, 423.
Griffiths, K., Davies, P., Harper, M. E., Peeling, W. B. and Pierrepoint, C. G. (1979). In *"Endocrinology of Cancer"*. (D. P. Rose, ed.), Vol. II, CRC Press, Inc., Florida.
Harper, M. E., Pierrepoint, C. G., Fahmy, A. R. and Griffiths, K. (1970). *Biochem. J.* **119**, 785.
Harper, M. E., Fahmy, A. R., Pierrepoint, C. G. and Griffiths, K. (1970). *Steroids* **15**, 89.
Hawkins, E. F., Nijs, M., Brassinne, C. and Tagnon, H. J. (1975). *Steroids* **26**, 458.
Hayward, J. (1970). In *"Hormones and Human Breast Cancer"*. Heinnemann, London.
Huggins, C. and Clark, P. J. (1940). *J. Expt. Med.* **72**, 747.
Huggins, C., Stevens, R. E. Jr. and Hodges, C. V. (1941). *Arch. Surg.* **43**, 209.
Huggins, C. and Hodges, C. V. (1941). *Cancer Res.* **1**, 293.
Hunter, J. (1786). *Bibliotheca Osteriana.* 1st Edition, 39.
Jones, V. (1970). In *"The Clinical Management of Advanced Breast Cancer"*, Second Tenovus Workshop. (C.A.F. Joslin and E.M. Gleeve, eds.), p. 24. Alpha Omega Publishing, Cardiff.
Leav, I., Morfin, R. F., Ofner, P., Cavazos, L. F. and Leeds, E. B. (1971). *Endocrin.* **89**, 465.
Maynard, P. V., Bird, M., Bash, P. K., Shields, R. and Griffiths, K. (1976). *Europ. J. Cancer* **14**, 549.

Nicholson, R. I. and Golder, M. P. (1975). *Europ. J. Cancer.* **11**, 571.

Nicholson, R. I., Golder, M. P., Davies, P. and Griffiths, K. (1976). *Europ. J. Cancer* **12**, 711.

Nicholson, R. I., Davies, P. and Griffiths, K. (1977). *Europ. J. Cancer* **13**, 201.

Nicholson, R. I., Davies, P. and Griffiths, K. (1977). *J. Endocrin.* **73**, 135.

Nicholson, R. I., Davies, P. and Griffiths, K. (1978). *Europ. J. Cancer* **14**, 439.

Nicholson, R. I., Syne, J. S., Daniel, C. P. and Griffiths, K. (1979). *Europ. J. Cancer* **15**, 317.

Nicholson, R. I. and Griffiths, K. (1980). *In "Advances in Sex Hormone Research"*. (J. A. Thomas and R. L. Singhul, eds.) Vol. 4. Urban and Schwarzenberg Inc.

Oshima, M., Wakabayashi, K. and Tamaoki, B. (1967). *Biochim. Biophys. Acta.* **137**, 356.

Poortman, J., Prenen, J. A. C., Schwatz, F. and Thijssen, J. H. N. (1975). *J. Clin. Endocr.* **40**, 373.

Powell-Jones, W., Jenner, D. A., Blamey, R. W., Davies, P. and Griffiths, K. (1975). *Biochem. J.* **150**, 71.

Powell-Jones, W., Davies, P. and Griffiths, K. (1975). *J. Endocrin.* **66**, 437.

Shimazaki, J., Kirihara, H., Yoshikazu, I. and Shida, K. (1965). *J. Med. Sci.* **14**, 313.

Teller, M. N., Kaufman, R. J., Stock, C. C. and Bowie, M. (1968). *Cancer. Res.* **28**, 368.

Wagner, R. K., Schulze, K. H. and Jungblut, P. W. (1975). *Acta Endocr.* (Kbh) Suppl. 193, Abst. 52.

Discussion

Catane: I think we should try to concentrate on why such promising agents like the nitrogen mustard derivatives of tamoxifen were relatively ineffective. We may be able to design more effective drugs by discussing why they were ineffective. Possibilities are that the drug hydrolyzes or is metabolized before arriving at the cell or maybe the compound doesn't enter into the cell. Dr. Griffiths, do you have any idea why this agent was ineffective?

Griffiths: We don't. We can imagine that compound 79792 does not bind to the receptor as well as does tamoxifen and that is why you would get a less effective action. At the present time we are trying to find out what the metabolism is of all these compounds.

Katzenellenbogen: You mentioned the blood levels of tamoxifen and its metabolites. Can you determine the tissue levels of these compounds?

Griffiths: Yes, the tissue levels are being determined but we don't have the tissue levels of the metabolites at the present time. The data, which I gave you, the 50,000/1 ratio in the tumor and in the nuclei of the tumor, were done last week. The metabolites are being measured to find out what in fact is in the nucleus. We know that there is about 15 ng/ml of the desmethyltamoxifen in the plasma and the preliminary data we have from the tissue levels would suggest that it is also present in the tumor in reasonable concentrations. ICI would tend to say that there is no hydroxytamoxifen in the plasma and that it does not play a role in the action of tamoxifen. Desmethyltamoxifen binds to the receptor but hydroxytamoxifen binds better.

Könyves: Do you have any clinical data on the ICI 85.966?

Griffiths: We don't have clinical data. There are several people in Britain who would like to use the compound in patients with breast cancer and see what happens. At the present time we do not have the material to give it to the patients.

Heuson: I would like to ask a question on the experiments you showed with estracyt. Can you tell us more about the patients who received the drug?

Griffiths: Yes, eight patients who had been on stilbestrol relapsed and were put on estracyt. We do have another study, where estracyt was used in the primary stage in twenty patients. Our feeling is that estracyt is something you use with recurrent disease.

Heuson: Yes, but if this compound hydrolyzes to such a proportion in the blood, the receptor would be saturated with a high affinity compound like estradiol which will saturate all the receptor sites.

Griffiths: We don't have any evidence at all that estradiol binds specifically to any receptor in prostatic tumor tissue. We can find estradiol receptors in stromal tissue but we do not have any evidence of an estradiol receptor in tumor tissue or hyperplastic prostatic tissue. We can obtain a good separation of the stroma from the epithelium and we can detect the extradiol receptor only in the stroma. These are data from the prostate of the dog.

Könyves: Do you think that there are some differences in the effects of various estrogenic drugs or estrogenic cytotoxic drugs on the differentiated versus the undifferentiated prostatic cancers?

Griffiths: At this particular time we tend to feel that those prostatic tumors, which are differentiated are the ones that respond to diethyl-stilbestrol readily. If the tumor is differentiated, it will respond to a change in hormone status and if it is not, the tumor is out of control. This means that this patient will soon be coming back with a recurrent disease. We have a new system in Cardiff which, I hope, will be developed in a short while. It consists of an ultrasound probe which scans around and measures the size of the prostate and determines also the changes in the shape and size of the prostatic tumors on treatment. This might help us a little more with this particular question that you just were asking.

Bloomer: Although sex steroid hormones are transported to all parts of the body via the blood stream, they stimulate only specific target cells containing receptors. A recently established *in vitro* line of human breast cancer cells containing estrogen receptor protein (MCF - 7) provides an opportunity to probe these sub-cellular hormone interactions. Tamoxifen is a non-steroid anti-estrogen that competes with estradiol for estrogen receptor protein. We speculated that ^{125}I-labeled tamoxifen (^{125}I-TAM) should be selectively cytoxic in MCF-7 cells and tested this hypothesis in MCF-7 and V-79 Chinese hamster cells.

We measured the cellular uptake of ^{125}I-TAM by both cell lines as a function of concentration in the media. An identical linear relationship between cellular uptake and media concentration for both cell lines suggests that entry of ^{125}I-TAM occurs by passive diffusion. Cytoxicity of ^{125}I-TAM was evaluated both as a function of media concentration and cellular concentration. ^{125}I-TAM is differentially cytotoxic to MCF-7 cells at concentrations between 1 and 20μCi/ml. Non-radioactive tamoxifen and Na^{125}I are both non-toxic at these levels of ^{125}I-TAM. When the surviving fraction is expressed as a function of cellular concentration, the D_{37} values are 1.5 and 0.5 pCi/ cell for V-79 and MCF-7 cells respectively.

These studies suggest that ^{125}I-TAM is selectively cytotoxic in cells containing estrogen receptors. The selective toxicity is presumed to result from translocation of the receptor ^{125}I-TAM complex from the cytoplasm to the nucleus.

Leclercq: I am not familiar with the V79 cell line. Do you have some data on the estrogen sensitivity?

Bloomer: The level of tamoxifen used in these experiments is not toxic in other cell lines. The V 79 is a Chinese hamster cell line. It is a standard mammalian cell line used in radiobiology labs. It has a different generation time than the MCF7 cell line, which has a much longer generation time; it is harder to grow. The estrogen receptor levels in this particular V79 cell line are about 2-4 fmoles per mg of protein and for the MCF7 it is about 60-65 fmoles per mg.

Paridaens: Did you measure the radioactivity of the nuclear fraction?

Bloomer: No, we haven't done that yet.

Paridaens: Because I don't agree with your conclusions. I would only conclude that your MCF7 is a hormone-sensitive line and the other is not.

Bloomer: My conclusion is that there is a difference in survival based on the cellular concentration. The reason for that we haven't proven, I agree.

Wittliff: Let me clarify. Did you say that at these levels of uniodinated tamoxifen the V79 cells survive?

Bloomer: Yes, uniodinated tamoxifen at the concentration used in these experiments is non-toxic to either cell line.
  The tamoxifen is simply a vehicle, or a carrier for getting a celltoxic isotope into a cell.

Wittliff: But in this cell line that hasn't much receptor it still gets in.

Bloomer: Previous workers have been using I^{125} uridine and I^{125} thymidine analogues. And that was the background information for us. I^{125} is extremely toxic to any cell that is rapidly growing. Unfortunately most cancer cells are not actively synthesizing: most of them are in a G_O stationary phase. That is why we tried to develop a different strategy to get I^{125} into the nucleus: we thought that the estrogen receptor might be a good way to do that. These are preliminary experiments that confirm, I think, our speculation or hypothesis.

Katzenellenbogen: I have a suggestion for two controls. This is very provocative work but I think you should do an experiment with a lipophilic iodinated compound which does not bind to the receptor, so that you can get it into those cells and just check whether the sensitivity to I^{125} is equivalent for both cells. Maybe you could use iodobenzene or something like that. You should also be able to demonstrate a protective effect with estradiol or with an excess of unlabeled tamoxifen at least if it is a receptor-mediated process. We should not forget all the biochemistry which has been done on receptors with competition experiments, when we do an uptake or a survival curve. If we really want to make receptor reagents we ought to be able to prove that they are working by receptor-mediated processes.

Borgna: Tamoxifen (Tam) is a triphenylethylene antiestrogen currently used in the treatment of breast cancer. But as yet, no data concerning the nature of the ligands bound to the estrogen receptor (ER), after *in vivo* Tam administration has been reported. Therefore we attempted to determine which compounds (Tam or metabolites) were concentrated at the ER sites. After *in vivo* administration of (^{3}H) Tam to immature female rats, the ethyl acetate extracts of plasma, cytosol and KCl-solubilized nuclear fraction of the uterus, were analysed by thin layer chromatography (TCL) (Borgna *et al.*, 1979). We found that polar metabolites of Tam were present in all the samples analysed (Fig. 1). Two of these polar metabolites (fractions no 2 and 5) represented the major part of the radioactivity in the uterine extracts, conversely Tam became negligible. These two polar metabolites appeared to occupy the uterine ER sites. This was based on the following evidence: 1) a progressive enrichment from plasma

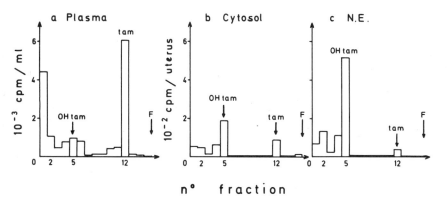

n°   f r a c t i o n

Fig. 1: Radiochromatograms of plasma, cytosol and nuclear fractions of rat uterus, after (^{3}H) tamoxifen administration.

Three immature female WISTAR rats, 20 days-old, received s.c. 15 μg of (^{3}H) tamoxifen (S. A. = 2.8 Ci/m mole). 8 h later, the plasma, the cytosol and the KCl-solubilized nuclear fraction (NE) of pooled uteri were prepared. The ethyl acetate-extracted radioactive compounds from plasmas and charcoal-treated (1h, 0°C) uterine fractions were analysed by TLC on silica gel plates.

Fraction no 1: deposit; fraction no 15: front of eluant (F).

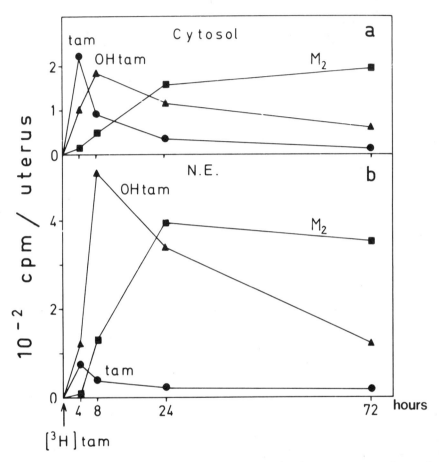

Fig. 2: Time-dependent variation of the charcoal-resistant concentrations of tamoxifen and of its main metabolites in uterine fractions:

The experiment described in Fig. 1 is performed for increasing periods of time after (^{3}H) tamoxifen injection. The radioactivity from uterine cytosol and nuclear extract (NE) found in fractions 2 (■); 5 (▲) and 12 (●) of TLC are represented.

to cytosol and nuclear fractions; 2) a saturable accumulation in uterine fractions; 3) a resistance to charcoal adsorption which was higher for polar metabolites than for Tam. The concentrations of these metabolites in uterine fractions varied according to time (Fig. 2). On the day following the injection a monohydroxy derivative of Tam (OH Tam in fraction no 5) was predominant. This metabolite has been identified by co-crystallisation with non radioactive OH

Tam until constant specific activity. On the two following days, the uterine content of OH Tam decreased while an unidentified (but probably hydroxylated) more polar compound (metabolite M_2 in fraction no 2) became predominant. Similar results were obtained in the male chicken liver. A high level of polar metabolites was found after an *in vivo* injection or an *in vitro* incubation of liver with (^{3}H) Tam. The OH Tam formed *in vitro* was the main compound bound to ER in a liver nuclear fraction. We therefore conclude that OH Tam is actually formed *in vivo* and retained at the ER sites in the rat uterus and chicken liver. Moreover this compound shows a much higher affinity for ER *in vitro* (Jordan *et al.*, 1977; Rochefort *et al.*, 1979; Nicholson *et al.*, 1979) and a much higher antiestrogenic activity *in vivo* as compared with Tam both in the rat uterus (Jordan *et al.*, 1977) and human breast cancer cells (Westley *et al.*). These data strongly suggest that *in vivo* Tam acts indirectly *via* hydroxylated metabolites.

Acknowledgments

We are grateful to Dr. Patterson and ICI Laboratories for providing us with (^{3}H) tamoxifen and hydroxytamoxifen. We thank Mrs. S. Ladrech for technical assistance. This work was supported by the Institut National de la Santé et de la Recherche Médicale and the Délégation Générale à la Recherche Scientifique et Technique.

References

Borgna, J. L. and Rochefort, H. (1979). *C. R. Acad. Sc.* in press.

Jordan, V. C., Collins, M. M., Rowsby, L. and Prestwich, G. (1977). *J. Endocrinol.* **75**, 305-316.

Nicholson, R. I., Syne, J. S., Daniel, C. P. and Griffiths, K. (1979). *Eur. J. Cancer* **15**, 317-329.

Rochefort, H., Garcia, M. and Borgna, J. L. (1979). *Biochem. Biophys. Res. Commun.* **88**, 351-357.

Westley, B. *et al.*, in preparation.

STEROIDAL ANALOGS OF NUCLEOSIDES AND NITROIMIDAZOLES AS POTENTIAL THERAPEUTIC AGENTS

J. E. VAN LIER

*Department of Nuclear Medicine
and Radiobiology,
Centre Hospitalier Universitaire,
Sherbrooke, Quebec, Canada*

Introduction

The major classes of anticancer chemotherapeutic drugs include alkylating agents, antimetabolites of nucleic acids, steroid hormones and antibiotics (Zubrod, 1974). Most of these drugs have undesirable side-effects due to their non-selective actions on both normal and tumor cells and must be given at high concentration to be effective. A similar problem exist with radiosensitizers, such as metronidazole and misonidazole. These products have been proposed as a means to increase the effectiveness of radiation therapy, however, their neurotoxicity at high doses restricts clinical use (Adams, 1979; Dische, 1979).

With a view to reducing the required doses of antitumor agents, attempts have been made to increase their specificity and cell-penetrating properties by coupling them to steroid hormones (Carroll, et al., 1972; Jones et al., 1971; Larionov et al., 1962; Schneider et al., 1966). Most of these earlier reported combination drugs were obtained via ester linkage of the steroid and cytotoxic moiety. Although in vivo testing was promising (Bogden et al., 1974), in vitro studies suggested that such complexes hydrolyse and that their effect may be attributed to the action of the individual chemical entities (Shepherd et al., 1974). In these earlier studies, no attention was given to the receptor affinity of the drugs. In view of the increased understanding of steroid structure-activity-affinity relationship, interest in this approach of drug design has been revived (Leclercq et al., 1976), and its potential has been discussed in detail (Lippman, *et al.,* 1978).

We have recently proposed steroidal pyrimidines as potential organ-selective agents for cancer chemotherapy (van Lier *et al.,* 1977). The products consist of steroids coupled *via* a C-N linkage with naturally occurring pyrimidines. As with conventional steroidal combination drugs, the steroid moiety should provide the desired organ specificity. However, steroidal pyrimidines differ from such drugs in that neither component is cytotoxic. Instead, the coupled products may behave as nucleoside analogs, with antitumor activity resulting from interference at the DNA duplication level.

We have began the synthesis of steroidal nitroimidazoles as potential site-selective radiosensitizers along similar lines. Among the most common sensitizers used in conjunction with ^{60}Co-radiation treatment are metronidazole and misonidazole (Adams, 1979). (Fig. 1) Both products feature nitroimidazole as the entity with electron affinity. This class of drugs sensitizes poorly oxygenated (hypoxic) tumor cells which might otherwise survive the radiation treatment. Although they have shown great promise in earlier clinical trials, their use is limited by adverse side-effects, including neurotoxicity (Dische, 1979). Coupling of hormonal steroids with nitroimidazoles may provide radiosensitizers which concentrate selectively in the tissue to be treated.

As a further extension of this project we are evaluating the use of the same steroid moieties as a carrier of the short-lived Technetium-99m isotope. Among the more than 1400 available radionuclides, ^{99m}Tc is one of the few which have found routine applications in clinical diagnosis. In addition to its attractive physical properties, e.g.

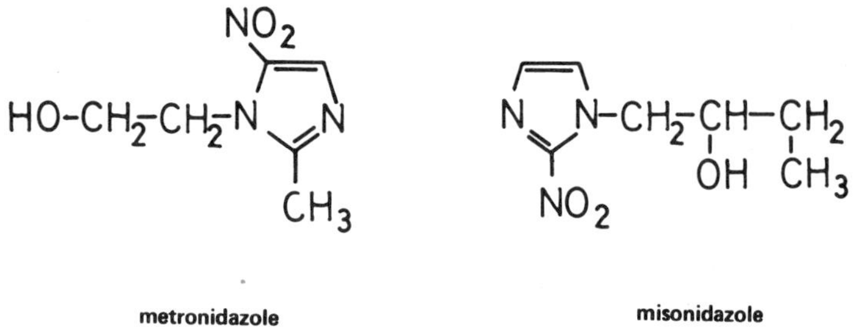

metronidazole   misonidazole

Fig. 1: Structures of two of the most common radio sensitizers.

half life of 6 hrs and single emitted γ of 0.14 MeV, the isotope can be supplied once a week as a ^{99}Mo/^{99m}Tc generator system to even the most remote hospital. From the generator Technetium is eluted as the pertechnetate ion (TcO$_4^-$) for the daily production of radiopharmaceuticals. The pertechnetate ion as such is useful for brain tumor and thyroid scanning, whereas the reduced form, Technetium oxide (TcO$_2$) may react rapidly with a variety of organic molecules to produce radiopharmaceuticals for nuclear medicine (Eckelman *et al.*, 1977). Iminodiacetate (IDA) has recently been demonstrated to be a strong chelator for TcO$_2$ and some N-substituted derivatives have been developed as useful scanning agents (Loberg *et al.*, 1978). On such accounts we are preparing steroidal-IDA derivatives which upon binding with ^{99m}Tc may provide diagnostic agents for hormone receptive tumors.

Synthesis

The three classes of agents, e.g. steroidal pyrimidines as nucleoside analogs, steroidal nitroimidazoles as electron-affinity radiosensitizers and steroidal ^{99m}Tc-chelators as γ-emitting scanning agents, share the same steroid intermediates. Coupling between steroids and pyrimidines or nitroimidazoles is accomplished by adapting general methods used in nucleoside chemistry (Watanabe *et al.*, 1974). The condensation involves conversion of the appropriate hydroxysteroid to the bromo- and mesyl-derivative followed by a reaction with the heterocyclic at elevated temperature to give C-N linkage. In the case of the pyrimidines the base is added as a persylitated product in the presence of a Friedel-Crafts (SnCl$_4$) catalyst (Niedballa *et al.*, 1974). A number of 3- and 21- substituted steroidal pyrimidines have been prepared in this manner (Hulsinga *et al.*,). Coupling of 21-hydroxysteroids through an ester linkage with nitrilotriacetate (NTA) to yield a N-substituted iminodiacetate (IDA) has also been accomplished. The formation of ^{99m}Tc-steroidal-IDA chelates has been postulated using established methods (Loberg *et al.*, 1978).

In an attempt to obtain steroid derivatives with a higher affinity for steroid receptors we are presently working on the synthesis of 6- and 16-substituted steroids. Some of the structures are given in Figure 2.

Biological testing

Receptor binding

Substantial affinity for specific hormone receptors is a basic requirement for a site-selective effect for either class of the steroidal agents

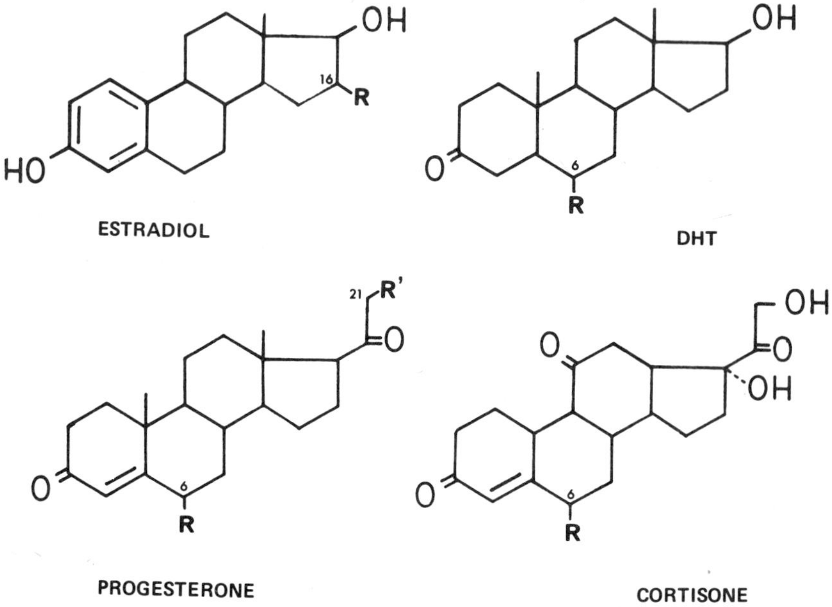

Fig. 2. Steroidal derivatives for which syntheses are in progress in our laboratory. The functional group R is a pyrimidine base (uracil, thymine) in the case
of nucleoside analogs; a nitroimidazole (5- or 4-nitroimidazole, 2-methyl-4-nitro-
imidazole) in the case of radiosensitizers; or a chelating moeity for ^{99m}Tc (N-
substituted iminodiacetate) in the case of scanning agents.

discussed in this article. Complete binding studies have been conducted for a series of 3- and 21-substituted steroidal pyrimidines only.
The 21-substituted progesterone derivatives showed weak affinity for
the androgen receptor whereas some of the 21-substituted corticoids
exhibited affinity for glucocorticoid receptor (Zava *et al.*, 1978). The
affinities are at least 1000 times less than the competing ^{3}H-steroids.
Similar results can be expected for either nitroimidazole or IDA
derivatives of this type. The 6- and 16-substituted steroids (Fig. 2)
with their bulky substituents remote from the functional groups of
the steroid molecule, may provide products with better receptor
binding properties.

Antitumor activity

The same series of 3- and 21-substituted steroidal pyrimidines were
tested *in vivo* in Fischer 344/CRBL rats bearing the 13762 mammary

adenocarcinoma and against the L 1210 lymphoid leukemia in female mice (van Lier *et al.*, 1978 & 1977). Only one product, the 3-uracil derivative of pregn-5-en-20-one (NSC-281832) gave presumptive activity in both screening tests. None of these products exhibited acute toxicity in CD-1 outbred albino female mice at 200 mg/kg. As suggested by Lippman *et al.*, (1978), future biological testing will first be done *in vitro*. The cell lines selected for the assessment of cytotoxic properties include the RBA and NMU lines from rat mammary tumors for androgen and glucocorticoid derivatives (Vignon *et al.*, 1979) and MCF_7 human breast cancer cell line for estrogenic compounds (Zava *et al.*, 1978).

Assessment of sensitizing activity

Steroidal nitroimidazoles with suitable affinity for steroid receptor can be tested for cytotoxic and sensitizing properties in the same cell lines as described above. As with established radiosensitizers, their action is expected to be mainly upon the dormant, radioresistant, hypoxic cells which are present at the interphase between well oxygenated regions of the tumor and the necrotic region (Thomlinson *et al.*, 1955). Accordingly, *in vitro* testing should be conducted on hypoxic cells. The sensitizing properties may be evaluated from radiation survival curves determined in the absence of oxygen and with various concentrations of the drug (Fig. 3). The percentage of cell survival after different doses of ^{60}Co-treatment may be deduced from the increase in DNA or cell content of the medium as a function of time post-irradiation. The radiosensitivity is defined as the slope of the linear portion of the semi-logarithmic plot of the surviving fraction (D_0). The effectiveness of the drug can be expressed by analogy to the oxygen enhencement ratio (OER), as the drug enhencement ratio (DER); representing the ratio of D_0 without or with the drug (Adams, 1979). It will be of particular interest to compare the DER value of such agents for different cell lines and to correlate them to cell receptor content.

Evaluation as scanning agents

N-substituted iminodiacetates are capable of forming stable dimers with ^{99m}Tc (Loberg *et al.*, 1978). In the case of the steroidal iminodiacetates, preliminary studies to prepare ^{99m}Tc-chelates have been conducted. Autoradiography of thin-layer chromatograms indicated the formation of several radioactive products and various purification procedures to obtain the steroidal-^{99m}Tc product are presently being assessed. In order to evaluate the tissue specificity of ^{99m}Tc-

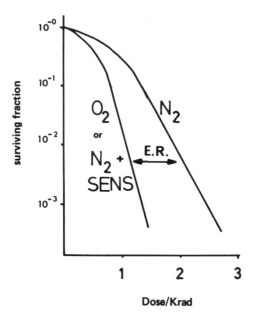

Fig. 3: Radiosensitizing properties of steroidal nitroimidazoles can be assessed from the survival curves of hormone receptive tumor cell lines. The effectiveness of the drug under hypoxic conditions mimics the oxygen effect and can be expressed as the enhencement ratio (ER). The drug enhencement ratio (DER) is defined as the ratio of the radiosensitivity of the hypoxic cells (D_O) without and with the drug. The radiosensitivity D_O inturn is defined as the slope of the linear portion of the semilogarithmic plot of the surviving fraction (Adams, 1979).

labeled products we selected as models Fischer 344/CRBL female rats with ant without the hormone sensitive 13762 mammary adenocarcinoma. These animals can be injected via the caudal vein and activity distribution can be followed by scintillation scanning with a Dyna-IV camara coupled with a Cybernex ordinator system (Cromemco). Selected images are registered on a magnetic disc, which allows for their presentation on a matrix of 128 by 128 points. The activity of each point is presented via a scale of 18 colors to cover an activity of 0-256 counts. In addition to the dramatic visualization of the scintillation scan, this technique allows for quantitative studies of the results.

Discussion

In our first approach to use steroids as site-selective carriers for therapeutic agents, we used steroid substrates which are chemically readily accessible at C_3 and C_{21} for C-N coupling with heterocyclics (van Lier *et al.,* 1978). The substituents selected were naturally occurring pyrimidine bases. Steroidal pyrimidines can be looked upon as nucleosides in which the steroid molecule is substituted for a sugar molecule and cytotoxic activities can be anticipated as a result of their nucleoside characteristics. Only weak affinity for steroid receptors was observed and the 3- and 21-substituted products lacked acute toxicity at 200 mg/kg doses (van Lier *et al.,* 1977; Zava *et al.,* 1978). We intend to evaluate some pyrimidine derivatives among the proposed C_6 and C_{16} substituted steroids, and to extend our program to include potential steroidal radiosensitizers and tissue imaging agents. Site-selective radiosensitizers are of particular interest since they might aid in killing hypoxic cells in hormone receptive tumors during radiation treatment. A model for hypoxic cells in tumors has been proposed by Thomlinson and Gray (Thomlinson *et al.,* 1955) and is depicted in Figure 4. Oxygen consumption by the viable tumor cells results in regions of low oxygen tension and may explain the formation of necrotic areas. Hypoxic cells are believed to exist at the interphase of the oxygenated and necrotic regions. These cells pose a greater hazard in view of their relatively greater resistance to radiation. Molecular oxygen has a high affinity for the solvated electrons liberated during radiolysis of tissue and the superoxyde thus formed may account for a number of secondary radical species which in turn destroy biomolecules vital to cell function. Thus, oxygenated cells are more sensitive to radiotherapy. Destruction of actively metabolising tumor cells by chemo- or radiotherapy permits hypoxic cells to be re-oxygenated thus providing a center for regrowth of the tumor (Adams, 1979). The drugs presently used in conjunction with radiotherapy lack site-specificity and have unde-

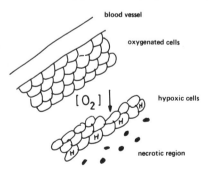

Fig. 4: The Thomlinson-Gray model for hypoxic cells in tumors (Thomlinson *et al.,* 1955). Oxygen diffuses from the blood vessel into the mass of tumor cells to sustain their viability. At about 150-200 microns away from the blood vessel little oxygen remains explaining the formation of necrotic regions. Hypoxic cells are believed to occur at the border of these regions.

sirable side-effects, particularly at the high concentrations required (Dische, 1979). By combining organ-specific steroid hormones with nitroimidazoles, the steroidal radiosensitizers promise to diminish both these problems. By a similar approach, N-substituted steroidal iminodiacetates, coupled with ^{99m}Tc, may provide useful scanning agents for visualisation of the metastases of hormone receptive tumors.

Acknowledgements

The author is grateful to the Medical Research Council of Canada and the Conseil de la Recherche en Santé du Québec for financial support.

References

Adams, G. E. (1979). In "Radiosensitizers of Hypoxic Cells" (A. Breccia, C. Rimondi and G. E. Adams, eds.) p. 13 and p. 245. Elsevier/North-Holland Biomedical Press., Amsterdam, New York, Oxford.

Bogden, A. E., Escher, H. J., Taylor, D. J., and Gray, J. H. (1974). Cancer Res. 34, 1627.

Carroll, F. I., Philip, A., Backwell, J. T., Taylor, D. J., and Wall, M. E. (1972). J. Med. Chem. 15, 1158.

Dische, S. (1979). In "Radiosensitizers of Hypoxic Cells" (A. Breccia, C. Rimondi and G. E. Adams, eds.) p. 221. Elsevier/North-Holland Biomedical Press., Amsterdam, New York, Oxford.

Eckelman, W. C., and Levenson, S. M. (1977). Int. J. Appl. Radiat. Isotop. 28, 67.

Hulsinga, E., Autenrieth, D., Ouellet, R., and van Lier, J. E., manuscript in preparation.

Jones, J. B., Adam, D. J., and Leman, J. D. (1971). J. Med. Chem. 14, 827.

Larionov, L. F., Degteva, S. A., and Lesnaya, N. A. (1962). Vopr. Onkl. 8, 12.

Leclercq, G., and Heuson, J. C. (1976). Current problems in Cancer 1, 1.

Lippman, M. E., Heuson, J. C., and Muggia, F. M. (1978). Cancer Treat. Rep. 62, 1267.

Loberg, M. D., and Fields, A. T. (1978). Int. J. Appl. Radiat. Isotop. 29, 173.

Niedballa, U., and Vorbruggen, J. (1974). J. Org. Chem. 39, 3654 and 3668.

Schneider, F., Hamsher, J., and Beyler, R. E. (1966). Steroids 8, 553.

Shepherd, R. E., Huff, K., and McGuire, W. L. (1974). J. Natl. Cancer Inst. 53, 895.

Thomlinson, R. H., and Gray, L. H. (1955). Brit. J. Cancer 9, 539.

van Lier, J. E., Kan, G., Autenrieth, D., and Hulsinga, E. (1978). Cancer Treat. Rep. 62, 1251.

van Lier, J. E. Kan, G., Autenrieth, D., and Nigam, V. N. (1977). Nature 267, 522.

Vignon, F., Chan, P-C., and Rochefort, H. (1979). Mol. Cell. Endocrinol. 13, 191.

Watanabe, K. A., Hollenberg, D. H., and Fox, J. J. (1974). J. Carb. Nucl. 1, 1.

Zava, D. T., and McGuire, W. L. (1978). Endocrinol. 103, 624.

Zava, T. D., McGuire, W. L., and van Lier, J. E. (1978). *J. Steroid Biochem.* **9**, 1155.

Zubrod, C. G. (1974). *Life Sciences* **14**, 809.

Discussion

Rousseau: Earlier work by van Lier *et al.* (1977) has shown that steroidal-pyrimidines prolong the survival of rats bearing a mammary adenocarcinoma. It was unlikely that the antitumor effect resulted from a breakdown of the drugs to give free steroid. A series of 3- and 21- substituted steroids was evaluated for their receptor binding properties (Zava *et al.*, 1978). No affinity for estrogen (ER) and progesterone (PR) receptors was observed while some of the products showed a weak affinity for androgen (AR) and glucocorticoid (GCR) receptors. As some mammary tumors contain GCR and since glucocorticoids stimulate mammary tumor virus production (Shyamala and Dickson, 1976), interaction of steroidal pyrimidines with GCR may influence development of such tumors.

This led us to investigate whether the 21-substituted steroids bound to the same site on GCR as the active glucocorticoids and whether such compounds were endowed with glucocorticoid activity. Experiments were conducted in rat hepatoma cells which, unlike the liver, contain only GCR and respond to glucocorticoids by induction of tyrosine aminotransferase (TAT).

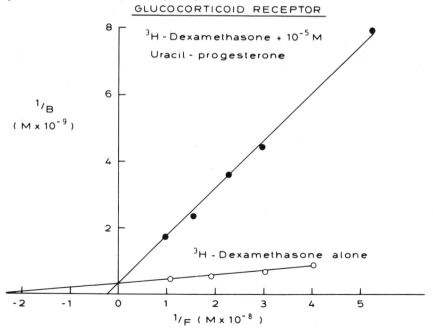

Equilibrium affinity constants (K_D, $0°C$) determined by competition with ^{3}H-dexamethasone in cell-free extracts were as follows:

Compounds	K_D (nM)
Progesterone	30
21-(thymine)-Progesterone	1695
21-(uracil)-Progesterone	1065
Cortexolone	70
17-Hydroxyprogesterone	175
21-(thymine)-17-hydroxyprogesterone	3000
Cortisone	745
21-(thymine)-Cortisone	2365

This is consistent with data obtained on rat liver (Zava *et al.,* 1978). Furthermore double-reciprocal plots suggested that competition takes place at the dexamethasone-binding site. Finally, 21-(uracil)-Progesterone at a concentration (10 μM) which did not induce TAT, inhibited by 25 % TAT induction by 25 nM dexamethasone. Consistent with their lower affinity for GCR, the other steroidal-pyrimidines did not influence TAT.

These results confirm that a pyrimidine base at C-21 does not prevent steroids from interacting, albeit with low affinity, with the glucocorticoid-binding site on GCR. However, this interaction does not elicit a glucocorticoid effect. This may have important implications if it is assumed that GCR must be bound by an agonist steroid in order to interact with DNA, a possible target for cytotoxic agents. Whether GCR binding and (or) antiglucocorticoid activity of steroidal pyrimidines is involved in the chemotherapeutic effect remains to be established.

Paridaens: Dr. Van Lier, it is known that technetium is a label for platelets and lymphocytes and I am wondering whether the technetium you fixed on the steroid did not exchange with these elements because then it would be a rather non specific labeling of inflamed tissue.

Van Lier: We are convinced that these compounds are stable. We did the excretion curves and they seem to bind irreversibly.

Paridaens: Yes, but the technetium could bind on the surface of the lymphocytes and platelets instead of on the receptor.

Van Lier: Yes, that is possible.

Katzenellenbogen: Do you have any evidence that your 5 FU conjugate would be cytotoxic by the same mechanism as 5 FU itself.

Van Lier: The funny thing is that they were not toxic. It was the free uracyl, the one substituted on the nitrogen which is normally, attached to the sugar, that had some effect on this *in vivo* tumor system. The 5 FU did not have any effect.

Katzenellenbogen: Are the *in vivo* animal systems you used sensitive to hormones?

Van Lier: This system is supposed to be responsive to estrogens but the last time that the number of receptors was determined in this tumor the concentration of receptor sites was about 3 fmoles per mg. This means that the receptor content is very low. We have not checked it, so we don't know how many receptors there actually were in this tumor line at the time of our experiment.

Katzenellenbogen: What concentrations of radiosensitizers are typically used? Do you have any idea of the cellular concentrations that are required?

Van Lier: Apparently the intracellular concentration of these nitroimidazoles is the same as the concentration in the blood. The concentration is extremely high. You cannot use them at that level because at that concentration they are neurotoxic. We thought that if we added some specificity to the nitroimidazole group we could lower this dose and get around the neurotoxic effect of these compounds.

Catane: Do you have any agent ready?

Van Lier: Not really, we are preparing one.

References

Shyamala, G. and Dickson, C. *Nature* **262**, 197-112 (1976).
Van Lier, J. G., Kan, G., Autenrieth, D. and Nigam, V. N., *Nature,* **267**, 522-523 (1977).
Zava, T. D., McGuire, W. L. and Van Lier, J. E., J. *Steroid Biochem.* **9**, 1155-1158 (1978).

THE FATE AND BIOCHEMICAL EFFECTS
OF ESTRACYT IN THE HUMAN AND BABOON

AVERY A. SANDBERG

Roswell Park Memorial Institute,
Buffalo, N.Y., U.S.A.

Advances in the synthesis of steroid conjugates with chemotherapeutic drugs as potential agents in the treatment of human cancer
are of relatively recent origin (Könyves *et al.*, 1975; Trams *et al.*,
1977). An underlying logic behind the synthesis of such conjugates
was based on the demonstration that certain tissues contain specific
receptors for steroid hormones (Sandberg *et al.*, 1970), particularly
those "target tissues" in which the steroids have a decided effect on
the anatomic integrity and function of the organ (Von Hoff *et al.*,
1977), e.g. breast, prostate, uterus, etc. These conjugates were conceived with the idea that by attaching a drug to a steroid hormone
(Fig. 1), the latter as part of its high affinity for and its association
with the intracellular receptor would carry the chemotherapeutic
drug "piggyback" into the cell, where it was hoped antitumor effects
would be produced either by the intact conjugate molecule or
following hydrolysis of the complex leading to release of the chemotherapeutic drug. Inherent in this concept is the assumption that
substitutions on the steroid molecule do not modify the following.
transport of the steroid in the blood and/or across cell membranes,
binding to plasma proteins and, most importantly, its interaction
with a specific receptor. Of crucial importance also is the necessity
of having the molecule remain intact while in the circulation, at
least in amounts sufficient to localize in the target organ (in this case

Abbreviations used: E_2 Estradiol-17β, E_1 Estrone, TeBG Testosterone binding
protein (globulin), i.v. intravenously, CCD Countercurrent distribution, T
testosterone, DHT Dihydrotestosterone, LHRH Luteinizing hormone releasing
hormone.

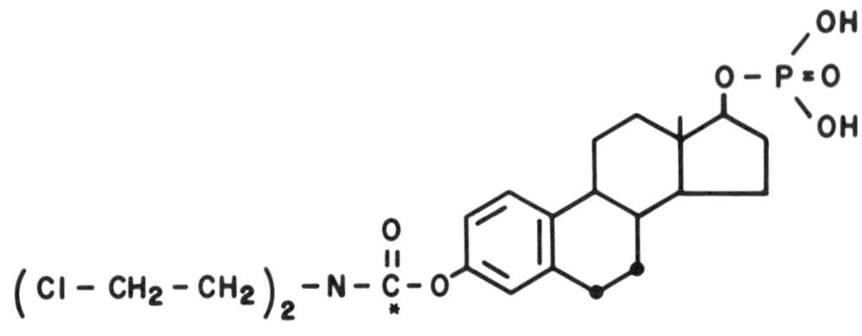

ESTRACYT

Fig. 1: Chemical formula of estramustine phosphate (estracyt) showing it to be an ester of a nitrogen mustard and E_2, the former being attached to the latter at position-3. A phosphate group is present at position-17. The drug consists of estradiol-3-bis(2-chloroethyl)carbamate-17-dihydrogen phosphate. For the drug to be effective it is thought that the phosphate group must be removed by phosphatase. The labeling of the drug is usually accomplished with ^3H at positions 6 and 7 of the E_2 moiety (shown by the dark circles) and that of the carbamate moiety by incorporating ^{14}C into one of the carbons (shown by the asterisk).

a tumor), rather than have it totally hydrolyzed, leading to separate activities of the individual compounds, i.e., the steroid and chemo-therapeutic drug, and, thus, possibly preventing the desired intra-cellular localization of the latter. The survival of the intact molecule in sufficient amounts may also depend on the mode and/or route of administration of the drug and in preclinical studies on the test animal used. In the case of estracyt, for example, it is readily hydro-lyzed in the circulation of the dog leading to toxic effects of the nitrogen mustard moiety, whereas the human and rat appear to hydrolyze the compound to a much lesser degree, resulting in the persistence of substantial amounts of unhydrolyzed compound in the circulation and, thus, in tissues.

That drugs may possibly be effective through binding to intra-cellular substances other than steroid receptors is a definite possibi-lity and one such example has been recently reported. Thus, it has been demonstrated that a binding protein, first found in the cytosol of the rat ventral prostate (Forsgren *et al.,* 1979 & 1978), with a high affinity for estracyt may play a role in the localization of the drug in that gland. This protein is probably akin to prostatein (Lea *et al.,* 1979), an α - protein (Shyr *et al.,* 1978) and a prostatic binding protein (Heyns *et al.,* 1978) described by others. The pre-sence of a similar protein in the human prostate has also been reported (Forsgren *et al.,* 1978). The relatively high affinity of this protein for and its specificity in binding the intact estracyt molecule may possibly be related to the antiprostatic effect of the drug.

Vexing has been the problem of finding an animal which could be used as a surrogate for the human, at least as far as the metabolism, fate and biochemical effects of estracyt were concerned. In our laboratory we chose the baboon on the basis of studies in which it was shown that the metabolism of a number of steroids (estrogens, androgens and progestational compounds) in the baboon was very similar to that of the human (Honjo *et al.*, 1976 & 1976, Ishihara *et al.*, 1975, Karr *et al.*, 1978, Yamamoto *et al.*, 1978). This was not true of a number of other animals investigated by us: rat (Sandberg *et al.*, 1970), rabbit (Sandberg *et al.*, 1970), sheep (Yamamoto *et al.*, 1978), dog (Yamamoto *et al.*, 1978) and rhesus monkey (Yamamoto *et al.*, 1978). Particularly disturbing was the range and difference in the biliary excretion of the various steroids (Sandberg *et al.*, 1970). In the human the biliary route is the major one for the excretion of estrogens but a minor route for most neutral steroids. None of the animals, except the baboon, resembled the human in the biliary excretion of steroids, e.g., in the rat all steroids are preponderantly excreted in the bile. Differences in the metabolism and/or conjugation of steroids among animals was another facet which ultimately led us to use the baboon for studies on estracyt metabolism, since this primate resembled the human in the metabolism of most steroids. Hopefully, data obtained in the baboon can be extrapolated to the human condition. Furthermore, the prostate of the baboon shares many features in common with that of the human, e.g, anatomic similarity, androgen and estrogen receptors and presence of TeBG (in plasma) (Karr *et al.*, 1979, 1978 & 1979, Müntzing *et al.*, 1976). Thus, my presentation will deal primarily with the metabolism and biochemical effects of estracyt in the human and to a lesser extent in the baboon; in the latter, studies not readily performed in the human can be accomplished (e.g., biliary excretion).

The metabolic fate of estracyt has been studied primarily by labeling the molecule with an isotope or isotopes (Fig. 1). Originally, only the steroid moiety was labeled with ^{3}H; under these circumstances the metabolism of estracyt was best compared to co-administered but differently labeled (with ^{14}C) E_2. This approach afforded a comparison of the excretion rate, fate and metabolic transformation and conjugation of the steroid released from estracyt with those of the co-administered free E_2. Subsequently, doubly labeled estracyt (^{3}H in the steroid and ^{14}C in the carbamate) afforded an opportunity to follow the fate of the total molecule, which was not possible when only the steroid was labeled. Under these circumstances the extent of hydrolysis and fate of the two moieties in estracyt could be ascertained.

Essential to the understanding of the fate of estracyt are the initial steps in its metabolism, which ultimately lead to either hydrolysis of the molecule and/or its excretion. These steps are shown in Figure 2 and indicate that dephosphorylation at the 17-position is the initial step. Apparently, dephosphorylation can be readily accomplished by most tissues, including the normal and abnormal human prostate (Fig. 3), and is probably not a limiting step in the metabolism and/or action of estracyt. In fact, dephosphorylation by plasma containing high levels of acid and alkaline phosphatases from a patient with carcinoma of the prostate has been demonstrated (Tritsch *et al.,* 1974). In all probability, the normal levels of these enzymes in blood are sufficient for such hydrolysis, though this has not been established with certainty. Following dephosphorylation, estramustine under- goes oxidation at position-17 of the estradiol-17β (E_2) moiety lea- ding to the appearance of compound 271, i.e., a conjugate of estrone (E_1) with the carbamate. The step involves the action of estera- ses present in a number of tissues, including the normal and abnor- mal prostate, resulting in the liberation of free E_1 (or E_2) and the nitrogen mustard. Much more is known of the metabolic fate of the

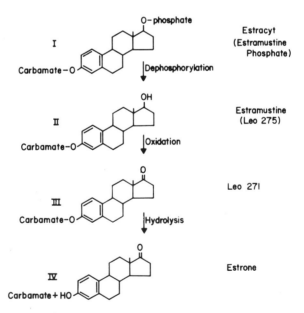

Fig. 2: Major initial pathways for the metabolism of estracyt (I). The first step usually involves removal of the phosphate leading to estramustine (II) (Leo 275), followed by oxidation at position-17 of the E_2 and resulting in Leo 271 (III). The next step is hydrolysis of the molecule resulting in the splitting of the carbamate from the estrogen, resulting in free nitrogen mustard and E_1.

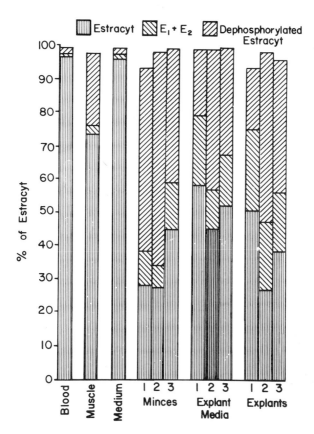

Fig. 3: Percentage of labeled estracyt dephosphorylated and hydrolyzed (shown as E₁ plus E₂) by various human fluids and tissues *in vitro*, including 3 adeno-carcinomas of prostate (Kadohama *et al.*, 1978). The latter were investigated as minces and explants in organ culture. Explant media were examined after the period of culture was completed. The stability of estracyt in blood and medium and its dephosphorylation and hydrolysis by prostatic tissue preparations are depicted.

steroid moiety than of the mustard (Figs. 4-10). Estradiol-17β or estrone join the general body pools of E_2 or E_1 (Fig. 6), these steroids are excreted preponderantly in the bile, followed by a substantial enterohepatic circulation with the conjugated metabolites ultimately reaching the urine but over a prolonged period of time (Sandberg *et al.*, 1970). As indicated, the fate of the carbamate is at the present essentially unknown. When the excretion of co-administered free E_2 is compared with that of the E_2 in the estracyt, the quantitative differences are remarkable (Figs. 4,5 & 8). At least 2-3 times more of the radioactivity of the free E_2 is excreted in the urine

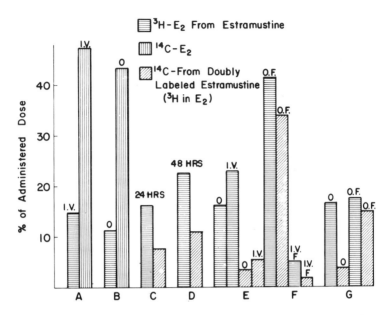

Fig. 4: Excretion of radioactivity in the urine of patients given radioactive estra-cyt or estramustine and free E_2. In A is shown the excretion in the first 24 hrs. following the i.v. administration of estramustine labeled with ^{3}H in the E_2 moiety and that of coadministered free E_2 labeled with [14]C (Kirdani *et al.,* 1975). The excretion of radioactivity associated with the free E_2 was more than 3-fold that originating from estramustine. In B is shown a similar study, but in which the compounds were given orally. In this case, the excretion of radio-activity associated with the administered ^{14}C-E_2 was 4-fold that of the coadmi-nistered estramustine. In C and D are shown excretions of radioactivity of doubly labeled estramustine given either orally or i.v. The excretion of the radioactivity associated with the estrogen moiety is similar to that shown in A and B, whereas that related to the nitrogen mustard is about half of that of the estrogen. In E and F are shown the urinary and fecal excretions of radioactivity following the administration, either orally or i.v., of doubly labeled estracyt to the same subject, but on two different occasions (Plym Forshell *et al.,* 1976) As in C and D, much less of radioactivity associated with the carbamate was excreted as compared to that of the estrogen. Also, the activity excreted in the feces (O.F.) is much higher following oral than the i.v. administration of the drug. In G is shown the excretion of radioactivity following the oral administra-tion of doubly labeled estracyt; the results are very similar to those shown in E, though the excretion in feces appears to be of a somewhat lower order of magnitude than observed in the study shown in F.

over a similar period of time, as that exhibited by the E_2 in the estracyt. This appears to indicate that either estracyt is sequestered in body compartments where the compound is not readily hydroly-zed and/or that it is excreted intact through the biliary route without

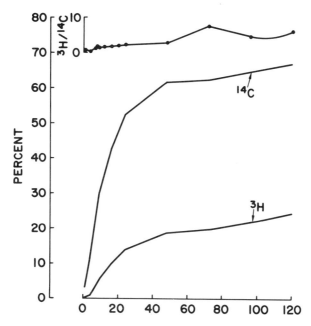

Fig. 5: Excretion (percent of administered dose) of radioactivity in urine of a subject after the i.v. injection of ³H-labeled estracyt (29.2 μCi) and ¹⁴C-labeled E_2 (5 μCi) (Kirdani *et al.*, 1975). The uppermost curve represents the isotope ratio in the various urine collections. The radioactivity of the free E_2 (¹⁴C) was excreted in much larger amounts than that of the E_2 in the estracyt.

subsequent absorption and/or hydrolysis. Were the latter to occur in the intestinal tract, the excretion would be similar to that of the administered free E_2, that has not been the case. The fate of estracyt, whether administered intravenously (i.v.) or orally, appears to be very similar (Fig. 4), though some quantitative differences exist, which will be discussed below.

Results obtained following the i.v. or oral administration of singly or doubly labeled estracyt confirm the persistence of the intact molecule in plasma (Figs. 11 & 12). Thus, Plym Forshell *et al.* (1976) found that the preponderant compound present in the plasma following the i.v. administration of labeled estracyt was either the unchanged drug or its dephosphorylated product, estramustine. No free E_2 could be observed with the methodology used. Following oral administration of estracyt to one patient, most of the radioactivity in the portal blood was present as estramustine; this was also true to a large extent in the general circulation. The authors indicated that their findings point to about 75% of the oral compound

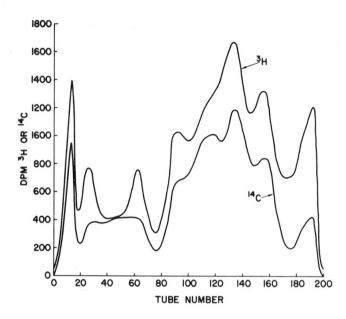

Fig. 6: Counter current distribution (CCD) of a urine of the subject of Fig. 5 (Kirdani *et al.*, 1975). Note the great similarity between the two curves beyond tube N. 80, indicating that the ^{3}H excreted (emanating from the labeled estracyt) is associated with released E_2 which has a CCD pattern very similar to that of the ^{14}C-E_2. The ^{3}H-peaks at tubes N. 24 and N. 64, not present in the ^{14}C-curve, probably indicate excretion of the intact estracyt molecule.

having been absorbed. This figure appears to me to be rather high, particularly in view of the substantial excretion of radioactivity in the feces of the subjects given the oral estracyt vs. that observed following the i.v. administration of estracyt (Fig. 4), unless the biliary excretion of estracyt and its metabolites following oral administration is much more extensive than that following i.v. administration, which appears to be unlikely. Gunnarson *et al.*, (1978) determined the metabolites of estracyt in the plasma in patients taking large doses of the drug. To a large extent, the authors confirmed the findings obtained with labeled estracyt, though they were able to show greatly increased levels of circulating E_1 and E_2, i.e., about 50-100 fold the level seen in normal men of the same age. However, the ratio of $E_1:E_2$ was much higher (more than 10) following estracyt administration than that seen under normal circumstances (a ratio of about 2). Again, the authors (Gunnarsson *et al.*, 1978) found large amounts of estramustine and compound 271 as the major circulating compounds following oral administration, pointing again to the intactness of the estracyt molecule absorbed from the gastrointestinal

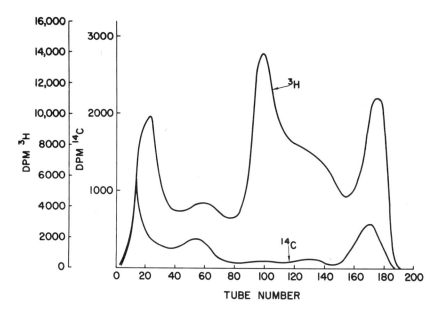

Fig. 7: CCD of a urine of a patient after the oral administration of doubly labeled estracyt (Kirdani *et al.*, 1975). The two largest ^{3}H peaks have no counterparts in the ^{14}C CCD curve and indicate that hydrolysis of the estracyt had occurred and that the excretion of radioactivity associated with E_2 was more marked and rapid than that of the ^{14}C from the carbamate moiety of the mustard. Location of ^{3}H and ^{14}C peaks in the same tubes point to intactness of the estracyt molecule. Though differing in detail, CCD patterns obtained on urines and biles of humans and baboons injected with either doubly labeled estracyt or estracyt labeled in the E_2 and co-administered with differently labeled free E_2, were similar qualitatively to those shown in Figs. 6 & 7, respectively, as was their interpretation.

tract; and explained the negligible estrogenic manifestations induced by estracyt, as compared to those seen following therapy with other estrogens, on the basis of this high $E_1:E_2$ ratio, i.e., that E_1 is known to have much less estrogenic activity than E_2 and that its competition with E_2 for receptor sites in tissues would also lead to a much reduced estrogenic effect than observed with E_2.

Yielding, in major respects, results similar to those discussed above, but in a few others disparate ones, was the study by Kadohama *et al.*, (1979). We found that following the administration of doubly labeled estracyt the major compounds in the blood 1/2 hr. later were compound 271 and estramustine, as well as large amounts of E_1 and E_2. Five hrs. later, compound 271 and estramustine still made up a substantial percentage of the circulating radioactivity; E_1 and E_2 also constituted a substantial part of that radioactivity.

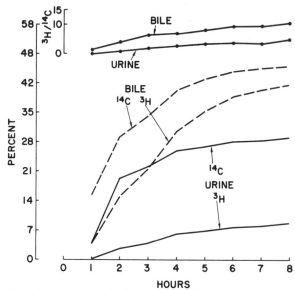

Fig. 8: Excretion (percent of administered dose) of radioactivity in bile and urine from a baboon injected with ^{3}H-estracyt and ^{14}C labeled free E_2 (Kirdani et al., 1975). As in the human, less of the radioactivity associated with the mustard moiety (^{14}C) was excreted than that of the E_2 moiety (^{3}H).

The ratio of $E_1:E_2$ was about 1, which contrasts with the findings of Gunnarson et al., (1978). However, in our case the compound was given to a patient who had not been on long-term therapy with estramustine, raising the possibility that such therapy may affect the metabolic pattern of estracyt by leading to a higher level of oxidation at the 17-position than in patients who had not received estracyt therapy. In fact, when a similar study (Honjo et al., 1976) was performed on a patient who had been on long-term estracyt therapy the results of Gunnarson et al., (1978) were confirmed, i.e., the ratio of $E_1:E_2$ was nearly 6:1 1/2 hr. after oral administration of estramustine and about 8:1 5hrs. later. The levels of compound 271 were 3-5 times that of estramustine at the times indicated. The observations of Fosså et al., (1977) confirm those of others, i.e., high levels of E_2 and total estrogens (20-50 fold of the pretreatment levels) were found in the plasma during and many weeks after cessation of estracyt therapy. The latter indicated to the authors that estracyt serves as a depot for these estrogens, in agreement with the findings originally reported from our laboratory (Kirdani et al., 1975). Incidentally, from the data of Fosså et al., (1977) it appears that the ratio of $E_1:E_2$ was 5-6 in most of the patients studied though it was not consistently so.

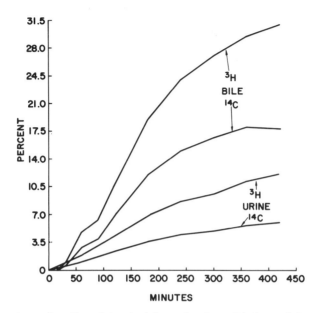

Fig. 9: Excretion of radioactivity in bile and urine of baboon injected with doubly labeled estracyt (Kirdani *et al.*, 1975).

Thus, the fate of estracyt administered to humans can be constructed, though somewhat incompletely, from the data presented so far. It would appear that the bulk of estracyt and/or its immediate metabolites (compound 271 and estramustine) are sequestered in body compartments from which the estrogen is released very slowly following intracellular hydrolysis. Some of the effects of estracyt may be due to localization of such intact molecules in specific cells, e.g., in cancer of the prostate (therapeutic effects), in the hypothalamus (inhibition of LH synthesis resulting in very low testosterone levels), in the liver (increased synthesis of TeBG and transcortin, etc.). Were the estrogen moiety of estracyt and related compounds to be released at a more rapid rate, one would expect it to join the estrogen body pool and be metabolized and excreted in a manner similar to that of E_2 or E_1; in fact, this has been shown to be the case for labeled E_2 released following i.v. or oral administration of estracyt. That E_2 and E_1 rise to very high levels in the plasma during estracyt therapy appears to be now well established, but this is accompanied by relatively mild estrogenic effects (Andersson *et al.*, 1977) which certainly are not as striking as those observed following the administration of other estrogens at much lower doses. This has been explained severally: 1. The high $E_1 : E_2$ ratio, with the former being a much less

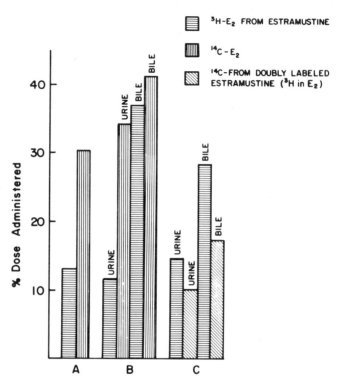

Fig. 10: Excretion of radioactivity in urine and bile of baboon injected i.v. with either doubly labeled estracyt (C) or ^{3}H-estracyt plus ^{14}C-E$_2$ (A&B) (Kirdani *et al.,* 1975). From A and B it appears that much more of the label from the free ^{14}C-E$_2$ was excreted in the urine (not bile) than that of the ^{3}H-E$_2$ in the estracyt. From C it is evident that much more of the E$_2$ moiety of estracyt is excreted both in bile and urine than of the mustard moiety.

potent estrogen than E$_2$,   2. The binding of the bulk of the circulating estrogens, particularly E$_2$, by the very high levels of TeBG (sex hormone binding globulin) (Fig. 13) and 3. A possible anti-estrogenic effect of intact estracyt, interfering with the metabolic effects of liberated E$_2$ and E$_1$ (Kirdani *et al.,* 1974).

That estracyt survives intact, at least as estramustine, following its oral administration is witnessed by the high levels of these two compounds in the peripheral circulation. Little is known about the fate of the released carbamate; its excretion appears to be even slower than that of the labeled steroid. There is always a possibility that it is metabolized to compounds which are eliminated and which cannot be readily measured, e.g., CO$_2$. Plym Forshell *et al.,* (1976) have suggested that the substituted carbamic acid may undergo ring

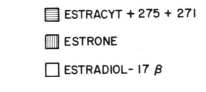

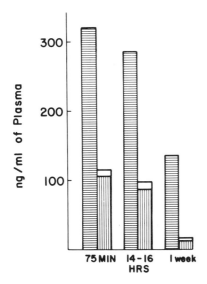

Fig. 11: Concentrations of various compounds in the plasma of subjects on estracyt therapy (ranging from 560-840 mg per day) with the levels shown being obtained after the last dose (Gunnarsson *et al.*, 1978). As can be seen, 75 min. following the oral administration of the last dose, the combination of estracyt, estramustine and 271 make up the bulk of circulating compounds, though the concentrations of E_1 and E_2 are also considerably elevated. A similar picture was seen 14-16 hrs. following the dose. One week after the last dose the levels of the intact compounds are still high, though the levels of the estrogens have dropped remarkably.

closure to N-β-chloroethyl-oxazolidone. However, if the carbamic acid is decarboxylated there will be no ring closure but a formation of the highly active N-β-chloroethyl-aziridine. The latter would be formed also if degradation of the ester occurred between the nitrogen and the adjacent carbon atom. No evidence exists for such degradation *in vivo*. It should be pointed out that the metabolic fate of the released E_2 or E_1 appears to follow that of systemic E_2 or E_1, at least as judged from the patterns of urinary excretion observed when estracyt is coadministered with labeled free E_2. Data also indicate absorption of the intact molecule of estracyt (or estramustine)

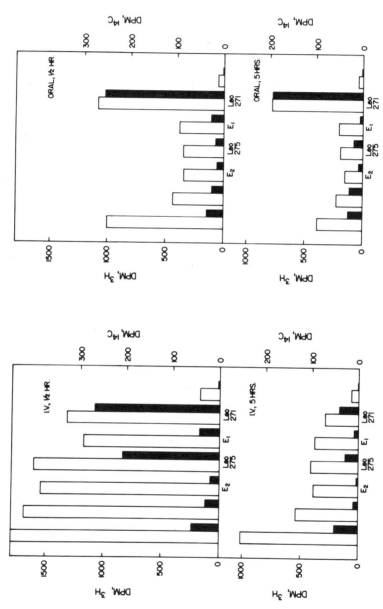

Fig. 12: Separation by thin layer chromatography of plasma extracts from patient following i.v. and oral administrations of estramustine labeled with ^{3}H (open bars) in the steroid and ^{14}C (closed bars) in the carbamate (Kadohama *et al.*, 1979).

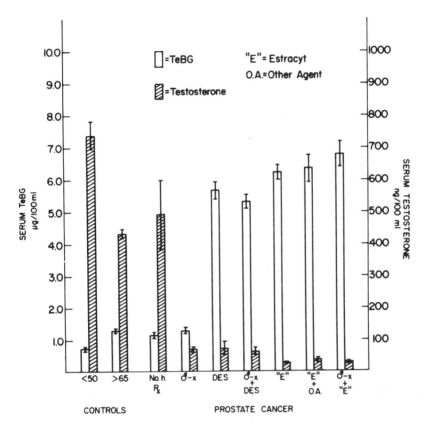

Fig. 13: Serum TeBG and testosterone levels of 2 male control and 7 prostate cancer groups (Karr *et al.*, 1979). Estrogenic effects of oral DES and estracyt therapy are illustrated by the marked elevation of serum TeBG and simultaneous depression of serum T. As indicated by us previously (Karr *et al.*, 1979), the lowest T levels and highest TeBG concentrations were observed in patients with cancer of the prostate who had been orchiectomized and received estracyt. Such a combination would lead to the lowest levels of unbound (active) T, which may play a role in the therapeutic effect of estracyt in this disease. ♂ - x = bilateral orchiectomy.

from the gastrointestinal tract, with a fate also different from that of coadministered free E_2. This difference not only applies to the much lesser excretion of the E_2 moiety in estracyt, but also to the persistence of large amounts of unhydrolyzed compound in the body and general circulation. Such differences are even more striking following the i.v. administration of estracyt plus free E_2.

Results obtained on the biliary excretion of estracyt and its metabolites in the baboon (Kirdani *et al.*, 1975), if they can be extrapolated

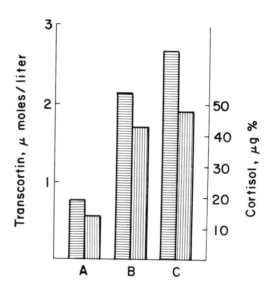

Fig. 14: Levels of transcortin and cortisol in patients with cancer of the prostate treated with estracyt for relatively long periods of time (Sandberg *et al.*, 1975). In A are shown the control levels and in B those obtained following therapy. It can be seen that the cortisol levels have risen considerably due to the binding of the steroid by the elevated transcortin. In C are shown transcortin and cortisol levels in patients on whom controls were not obtained and who had been on estracyt therapy. The results are similar to those in groups B and C.

to the human, indicate that though a substantial amount is excreted in the bile (about 35% of the administered dose), nearly 50% of the radioactivity cannot be accounted for and is probably related to the sequestration mentioned above (Fig. 16). That this probably also occurs in the human is indicated by the very low urinary excretion of radioactivity following oral or i.v. administration of labeled estracyt; for were large amounts to be excreted in the bile one would expect hydrolysis of the estracyt to have occurred prior to that event and to be accompanied by high levels of urinary excretion of the estrogen moiety and its metabolites. In other words, unless the intact estracyt molecule is excreted in the bile and is subsequently involved in a

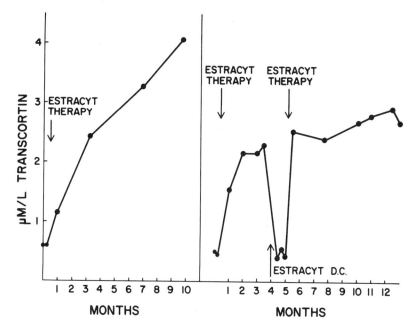

Fig. 15: Plasma transcortin levels in 2 patients following estracyt therapy (Sandberg *et al.,* 1975). In patient at left transcortin rose from normal to very high levels following therapy (4 micromoles). Patient depicted on right was started on estracyt, following which transcortin levels rose from normal to more than 2 micromoles. Because of severe nausea, the drug was stopped and transcortin levels returned to normal concentrations within two weeks after cessation of the drug. When estracyt was restarted one month later, transcortin levels again rose in response to therapy. Similar results have been obtained with serum TeBG. Failure of the levels of these proteins to rise has invariably indicated failure of the patients to take the drug and, thus, measuring the transcortin or TeBG levels may be used to monitor patients on estracyt.

very efficient and protracted enterohepatic circulation (for which there is no evidence), it would appear that, though a significant amount of estracyt and its metabolite are excreted in the bile, it still leaves unaccounted for a significant portion of estracyt, which is probably sequestered in compartments other than the liver and enterohepatic circulation.

That some of the metabolic effects of estracyt, and some of these may undoubtedly be related to its therapeutic effects, are mediated through the liberated estrogens, either intracellularly and/or released into the general circulation, is witnessed by a large array of changes similar to those induced by administered estrogens (Fig. 17). These include definite depression in the levels of the following in patients with prostate cancer: 17-hydroxyprogesterone, testosterone, DHT,

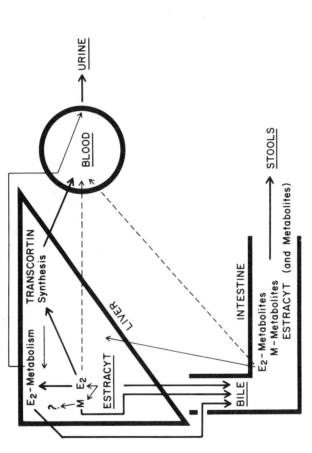

Fig. 16: Schematic presentation of fate of estracyt and its possible mechanism of raising plasma transcortin (or TeBG) levels (Sandberg *et al.*, 1975). The drug is shown to concentrate primarily in liver where it is hydrolyzed into its constituent E_2 and mustard (M). E_2 is then capable of inducing increased transcortin synthesis in liver cells, following which the E_2 is metabolized and conjugated in liver (E_2-Metabolism) without leaving that organ. Some of the conjugated metabolites of E_2 are then excreted in urine following their entry into blood, but bulk is excreted into the bile (E_2-metabolites). The latter, after entering the intestinal tract, are involved in an enterohepatic circulation. Broken lines point to possiblity of E_2 appearing in blood in high concentrations, for example, if the liver is incapable of effectively metabolizing released E_2 or due to excess hydrolysis of the drug with the result that some E_2 escapes from the liver into the circulation. The exact fate and metabolism of mustard moiety (M and M-metabolites) following hydrolysis in the liver are unknown.

FSH and LH (Jönsson *et al.*, 1975; Kirdani *et al.*, 1975). Accompanying these decreases are elevated levels of cortisol (due to increased concentrations of transcortin in the plasma (Figs. 14 & 15) and prolactin. In addition, decreased concentrations of pregnenolone and DHA were also found (Jönsson *et al.*, 1975). Other systemic effects in the human include a decrease of antithrombin III (Blombäck *et al.*, 1978), reduction in serum colesterol and an increase in serum phospholipids (Gustafson *et al.*, 1977). In aged males, the administration of estracyt (as well as estrogens) did not change carbohydrate metabolism, but did produce an increase in adipose tissue of lipoprotein lipase (Gustafson *et al.*, 1977).

In green monkeys the administration of estracyt led to markedly decreased levels of testosterone (pretreatment 698 ± 18 ng%; after 2 weeks of estracyt, 283 ± 61 ng%) (McMillin *et al.*, 1977). However, 2 months after therapy the testosterone levels returned to normal. The administration also led to increased transcortin levels and failure of the animals to respond to intravenously administered LHRH. No effect on the size of the testes or response of the pituitary adrenal axis was observed.

In the human prostate estracyt can displace about 50% of labeled E_2 bound (ca. 2 femtomoles/mg protein) by the cytosol of BPH prostate and over 70% of similar preparations obtained from cancerous tissue (Nilsson *et al.*, 1976). Similar results were obtained when DHT was used as a competitor. On the other hand, the binding of DHT by the same preparation (*ca.* 40 femtomoles/mg protein) was slightly affected by estracyt (less than 20% reduction), whereas E_2 competed very effectively with the bound DHT, raising the suspicion that the authors may have been studying primarily binding by TeBG. In the baboon the administration of estracyt has been shown to decrease zinc concentration, arginase and 5α-reductase activity in the prostate (McMillin *et al.*, 1977).

Attempts to demonstrate inhibition by estracyt of E_2 binding by estrogen receptor in the cytosol of human breast cancer tissue revealed little interference with such binding when incubated at 18°C for 30 min. (Leclercq *et al.*, 1976 & 1976). However, after 18 hrs. of incubation approximately 15% inhibition was observed, probably due to hydrolysis of the estracyt with resultant competition between the released E_2 with the labeled E_2. However, to suggest, as the authors did, that estracyt is probably not significantly concentrated by the estrogen target tissues such as mammary cancer and that, therefore, the drug is unlikely to be very valuable in the treatment of breast cancer through a specific mechanism involving concentration by the estrogen receptors appears to me to be some-

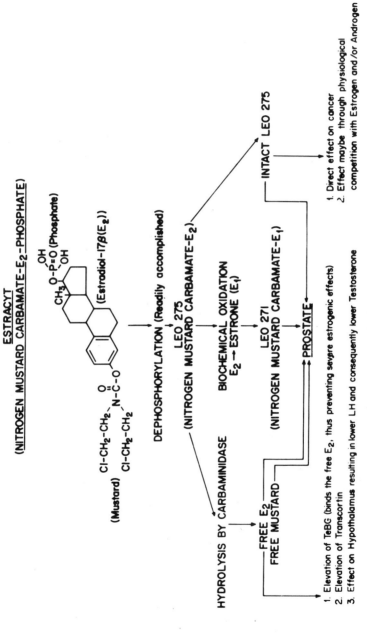

Fig. 17: (legend opposite)

what premature, since other avenues for effectiveness of the drug may be available and operative, without involving an estrogen receptor. In a recent report (Müntzing *et al.*, 1979) rat mammary tumors

Fig. 17: Schematic presentation of the fate, metabolic effects and mechanism of action (in cancer of the prostate) of estracyt and/or its products (Kadohama *et al.*, 1979).

By proceeding from top to bottom of the figure, the following important events relative to estracyt should be noted:

A. Dephosphorylation of estracyt with removal of the phosphate group at position-17 is readily accomplished in almost all body tissues and fluids, yielding estramustine.

B. Three different fates may then occur to estramustine: 1. Hydrolysis into its two constituents, i.e., E_2 and the nitrogen mustard (left side of figure); this apparently involves a relatively minor portion of estracyt during the initial 24-48 hrs. following i.v. or oral administration; 2. Oxidation of the E_2 moiety of estramustine, leading to oxidized estramustine (Leo 271) shown in the center of the figure. This and the preceding compound (Leo 275) are sequestered in body compartments, possibly including the prostate, from which they are very slowly excreted over a period of weeks to months following hydrolysis of the molecule; 3. Direct access of estramustine to tissues, including the prostate, shown on the right side of the figure; and 4. The events in 1. and 3. can all take place in the prostate.

C. Systemically liberated E_2 leads to the following: 1. Elevation of plasma TeBG, which binds to bulk of circulating E_2 and testosterone (T), thus, possibly preventing excessive estrogenic effects. 2. Elevation of plasma transcortin and cortisol concentrations due to the binding of the latter by the former, i.e., the very high levels of transcortin lead to elevated *total* plasma cortisol levels due to the binding of the steroid by the plasma protein; the elevated free (active) cortisol, leads to a partial "medical adrenalectomy,, resulting from suppression of ACTH release by the pituitary and, thus, in decreased secretion of adrenal androgens (and other steroids), which also may play a role in the effectiveness of the drug in cancer of the prostate; 3. Decreased circulating LH, probably through effects at the pituitary-hypothalamic level, leading to decreased T production; and 4. Possible direct effect on the prostate through the interaction of estracyt with the estracyt binding protein.

D. The liberated nitrogen mustard may have a direct effect on the prostate and other tissues following hydrolysis of the estracyt.

E. Intact estramustine and possibly its oxidized form (Leo 271) may compete physiologically with androgens and/or estrogens in the prostate, an effect depending on concentration of the compound in the tissue. Also, estramustine may have a direct effect on cancer cells of the prostate through a number of mechanisms (Fosså *et al.*, 1976; Kjaer *et al.*, 1975). The lack of outstanding estrogenic effects, particularly gynecomestia, in patients receiving estrogens may be due to a number of factors illustrated in the figure, including the high levels of TeBG which bind the circulating E_2 and E_1, the fact that most of the liberated E_2 is oxidized to E_1 resulting in rather high ratio ($> 5:1$) of $E_1:E_2$ as compared to a ratio of less than 2 under normal circumstances, and the possibility that estramustine may act as an antiestrogen and prevent the metabolic effectiveness of liberated E_1 and E_2.

induced by 7,12-dimethylbenz (α) anthracene showed a definite concentration of estramustine (doubly labeled) but no free E_2. The uptake of the drug in the tumors was paralleled by dose-dependent retardation of tumor growth and a prevention of tumor number increase. Estracyt also retarded the growth of mammary tumors resistant to treatment with E_2; the authors concluded that estracyt has a greater effect on tumor growth in this particular system than do estrogens.

A study in which estracyt at a dose of 420 mg daily was given to 44 postmenopausal women with very advanced breast carcinoma indicates that the drug may be of some value in this disease (Alexander *et al.*, 1979). Seventeen of the patients had an objective response and a marked or complete alleviation of symptoms, 4 others had useful symptomatic response and no beneficial effect was observed in the remaining cases. Apparently, estrogen receptor status and age within the postmenopausal group seemed to have no bearing on the clinical results. Except for nausea, the side effects were minimal. No bone marrow depression was seen, as has been the experience in patients with cancer of the prostate. Changes in acute phase reactant proteins suggested to the authors that part of the estracyt was hydrolyzed in the liver liberating E_1, whereas the low incidence of vaginal hemorrhage and evidence for recalcification of bony metastases indicated that estracyt may behave more as an antiestrogen than an estrogen and have definite antimitotic activity.

In a woman with breast cancer, who had been on estracyt therapy, following administration of the doubly labeled drug, significant concentrations of both labels were present in the breast cancer, as well as in tumor present in axillary lymph nodes, possibly indicating localization of the intact molecule (unpublished observations). In pectoralis muscle and normal breast tissue only the radioactivity of the estrogen moiety was found.

In summary, then, it appears that in the human and baboon the fate of the estrogen moiety released through hydrolysis of estracyt has a fate similar to that of systemic E_2, that most of the estracyt is sequestered intactly in body compartments where it is only slowly hydrolyzed, and that the anti-tumor effects of estracyt may, in fact, be partly due to this sequestration in organs with high affinity for the drug (e.g., cancer of the prostate). The fate of the carbamate moiety is essentially unknown.

Most of the metabolic effects of estracyt are due to the released E_2, either acting intracellularly at the site of its release or as a result of its joining systemic E_2. Anti-tumor activity may be ascribed to intact estracyt or its metabolites, to E_2 effects and, probably, to the released carbamate moiety.

References

Alexander, N. C., Hancock, A. K., Masood, M. B., Peet, B. G., Price, J. J., Turner, R. L., Stone, J., and Ward, A. J. (1979). *Clin. Radiol.* 30, 139.

Andersson, L., Edsmyr, F., Jönsson, G., and Könyves, I. (1977). *In "Recent Results in Cancer Research"* (E. Grundmann and W. Vahlensieck, eds), p. 73. Springer-Verlag Berlin Heidelberg, New York.

Blombäck, M., Edsmyr, F., Kockum, C., and Paul, C. (1978). *Urol. Res.* 6, 95.

Forsgren, B., Björk, P., Carlström, K., Gustafsson, J-A., Pousette, A., and Högberg, B. (1979). *Proc. Natl. Acad. Sci.* (USA) 76, 3149.

Forsgren, B., and Högberg, B. (1978). *Acta Pharm. Suec.* 15, 23.

Fosså, S. D., Fosså, J., and Aakvaag, A. (1977). *J. Urol.* 118, 1013.

Fosså, S. D., and Miller, A. (1976). *J. Urol.* 115, 406.

Gunnarsson, P. O., Nilsson, T., and Forshell, G. P. (1978). *Urol. Res.* (In press).

Gustafson, A., Nilsson, S., Persson, B., Tisell, L.-E., Wiklund, O., and Ohlson, R. (1977). *Invest. Urol.* 15, 220.

Heyns, W., Peeters, B., Mous, J., Rombauts, W., and DeMoor, P. (1978). *Eur. J. Biochem.* 89, 181.

Honjo, H., Ishihara, M., Osawa, Y., Kirdani, R. Y., and Sandberg, A. A. (1976). *Steroids* 27, 79.

Honjo, H., Ishihara, M., Osawa, Y., Kirdani, R. Y., and Sandberg, A. A. (1976). *Endocrinology* 99, 1054.

Ishihara, M., Osawa, Y., Kirdani, R. Y., and Sandberg, A. A. (1975). *Steroids* 25, 829.

Ishihara, M., Osawa, Y., Kirdani, R. Y., and Sandberg, A. A. (1975). *J. Steroid Biochem.* 6, 1213.

Jönsson, G., Olsson, A. M., Luttrop, W., Cekan, Z., Purvis, K., and Diczfalusy, E. (1975). *Vitam. Horm.* 33, 351.

Kadohama, N., Kirdani, R. Y., Murphy, G. P., and Sandberg, A. A. (1978). *J. Urol.* 119, 235.

Kadohama, N., Kirdani, R. Y. Madajewicz, S., Murphy, G. P., and Sandberg, A. A. (1979). *NY State J. Med.* 79, 1005.

Karr, J. P., Wajsman, Z., Madajewicz, S., Kirdani, R. Y., Murphy, G. P., and Sandberg, A. A. (1979). *J. Urol.* 122, 170.

Karr, J. P., Wajsman, Z., Kirdani, R. Y., Murphy, G. P., and Sandberg, A. A. (1979). *J. Urol.* (In press).

Karr, J. P., Kirdani, R. Y., Murphy, G. P., and Sandberg, A. A. (1978). *Arch. Androl.* 1, 123.

Karr, J. P., Kirdani, R. Y., Murphy, G. P., and Sandberg, A. A. (1979). *Arch. Androl.* 2, 123.

Karr, J. P., Sufrin, G., Kirdani, R. Y., Murphy, G. P., and Sandberg, A. A. (1978). *J. Steroid Biochem.* 9, 87.

Kirdani, R. Y., Müntzing, J., Varkarakis, M. J. Murphy, G. P., and Sandberg, A. A. (1974). *Cancer Res.* 34, 1031.

Kirdani, R. Y. Mittelman, A., Murphy, G. P., and Sandberg, A. A. (1975). *J. Clin. Endocrinol. Metab.* 41, 305.

Kjaer, T. B., Nilsson, T., and Madsen, P. O. (1975). *Urology* 5, 802.

Könyves, I., and Liljekvist, J. (1975). *In "Biological Characterization of Human Tumours"* , Excerpta Medica International Congress Series No. 375, p. 98. Copenhagen.

242   A.A. Sandberg

Lea, O. A., Petrusz, P., and French, F. S. (1979). *J. Biol. Chem.* **254**, 6196.
Leclercq, G., Deboel, M.- C., and Heuson, J.- C. (1976). *Int. J. Cancer* **18**, 750.
Leclercq, G., Heuson, J.- C., and Deboel, M.- C. (1976). *Europ. J. Drug. Metab. Pharmacokinet.* **1**, 77.
McMillin, J. M., Seal, U. S., and Doe, R. P. (1977). *Invest. Urol.* **15**, 151.
Müntzing, J., Varkarakis, M. J., Yamanaka, H., Murphy, G. P., and Sandberg, A. A. (1974). *Proc. Soc. Exp. Biol. Med.* **146**, 849.
Müntzing, J., Myhrberg, H., Saroff, J., Sandberg, A. A., and Murphy, G. P. (1976). *Invest. Urol.* **14**, 162.
Müntzing, J., Jensen, G., and Högberg, B. (1979). *Acta Pharmacol. Toxicol.* **44**, 1.
Nilsson, I., Liskowski, L., and Nilsson, T. (1976). *Urology* **8**, 118.
Nilsson, T., and Müntzing, J. (1973). *Scand. J. Urol. Nephrol.* **7**, 18.
Plym Forshell, G., Müntzing, J., Ek, A., Lindstedt, E., and Dencker, H. (1976). *Invest. Urol.* **14**, 128.
Sandberg, A. A., and Gaunt, R. (1976). *Semin. Oncol.* **3**, 177.
Sandberg, A. A., Slaunwhite, W. R., Jr., and Kirdani, R. Y. (1970). *In "Metabolic Hydrolysis"* (W. Fishman, ed), p. 123. Academic Press, New York.
Sandberg, A. A., Rosenthal, H., Mittelman, A., and Murphy, G. P. (1975). *Urology* **6**, 17.
Shyr, C.- I., and Liao, S. (1978). *Proc. Natl. Acad. Sci. USA* **75**, 5969.
Trams, G., and Urban, M.v. (1977). *Z. Krebsforsch.* **89**, 321.
Tritsch, G. L., Shukla, S. K., Mittelman, A., and Murphy, G. P. (1974). *Invest. Urol.* **12**, 38.
Von Hoff, D. D., Rozencweig, M., Slavik, M., and Muggia, F. M. (1977). *J. Urol.* **117**, 464.
Yamamoto, Y., Manyon, A., Kirdani, R. Y., and Sandberg, A. A. (1978). *Steroids* **31**, 711.
Yamamoto, Y., Manyon, A. T., Osawa, Y., Kirdani, R. Y., and Sandberg, A. A. (1978). *J. Steroid Biochem.* **9**, 751.
Yamamoto, Y., Peric-Golia, L., Osawa, Y., Kirdani, R. Y., and Sandberg, A. A. (1978). *Steroids* **32**, 373.
Yamamoto, Y., Osawa, Y., Kirdani, R. Y., and Sandberg, A. A. (1978). *Steroids* **31**, 233.

Discussion

Paridaens: I would like to ask two questions. How did you assay TeBG and does estracyt bind to TeBG?

Sandberg: For the determination of TeBG we used a column and estracyt does not bind to TeBG. There is no circulating protein that I know of, to which estracyt or estramustine binds.

Könyves: What is the situation if you give only estradiol?

Sandberg: If you give estradiol most of the estrogenic compound you find in the blood is estradiol. We get the impression that most of the estrogenic effects that we see may be due to the intracellular splitting of the molecule and the effects of estrogens manifesting themselves at that site. For example the very high levels of transcortin may be due to the fact that when the molecule gets into the liver it is hydrolyzed and before the estrogen is metabolized it has a chance to stimulate transcortin synthesis. However, we don't see gynlcomastia in these patients. Most of the toxic effects are gastrointestinal.

Wittliff: But you have taken isolated prostate explants and studied the metabolism of estramustine phosphate and it is not all hydrolyzed as I remember.

Sandberg: Yes, but these are 1 hour incubations.

Wittliff: But I mean from published data from your lab.

Sandberg: I could not tell you, maybe Dr. Forsgren will present some data on that.

Wittliff: I am wondering if that is part of the mechanism of why it has such a long half life.

Sandberg: You must realize that 50% of extracyt is not localized in the prostate. So you must look to other organs.

Heuson: All this is based on the assumption that estracyt will act on cancer of the prostate when other estragons or other treatments fail. It is difficult to say that a patient with cancer of the prostate, who is resistant to DES will react to estracyt. The only way to do the experiment is to randomize the patients and treat one group with DES and the other with estracyt and I don't know of any published report that shows such evidence.

Sandberg: Well, there is such evidence. The National Prostatic Cancer project has in fact exactly done what you just said. These data will be published in the near future. Maybe Dr. Catane can tell us more about these studies.

Catane: In the National Prostatic Cancer project the patients were randomized between estracyt treatment and conventional therapy. I don't know the exact figures but there was a clear advantage in giving estracyt instead of estrogens.

INTERACTION OF ESTRAMUSTINE,
A NITROGEN MUSTARD DERIVATIVE OF ESTRADIOL-17β, AND RELATED COMPOUNDS WITH THE PROSTATE

BJOERN FORSGREN, PER BJOERK, KJELL CARLSTROEM,
JAN-AKE GUSTAFSSON, BERTIL HOEGBERG, AND AKE POUSETTE

AB Leo Research Laboratories,
Helsingborg, Department of Chemistry, Department of Medical Nutrition
and Department of Pharmacology, Karolinska Institutet,
Hormone Laboratory, Sabbatsberg Hospital, Stockholm, Sweden

The discovery of selective accumulation of steroids in special "target" tissues offered a rational approach for utilizing estrogens and other steroid hormones as carriers for cytotoxic agents. In 1961 a cancer chemotherapy program including syntheses of several types of complexes between steroids and alkylating agents was started at AB Leo Research Laboratories, Helsingborg, Sweden (Könyves *et al.*, 1976). One of the compounds synthesized was estramustine phosphate, a nornitrogen mustard carbamate derivative of estradiol-17β esterified with phosphoric acid to achieve water solubility (Fig. 1). Estramustine phosphate was introduced as a therapeutic agent in the treatment of prostatic carcinoma in 1966 (Jönsson *et al.*, 1977). In order to understand the action of this compound in prostate tissue we have studied the uptake, metabolism, and binding of estramustine phosphate and/or its metabolites in rat and human prostate.

In distribution studies in rats Plym-Forshell and Nilsson (Plym Forshell *et al.*, 1974) using labeled compounds (1-10 mg/kg body weight) found considerably higher levels of radioactivity in the ventral prostate gland after intravenous administration of estramustine phosphate than after administration of estradiol-17β phosphate or estradiol-17β. The main metabolite of estramustine phosphate in the ventral prostate was identified as its dephosphorylated congener estramustine (Fig. 1). Høisaeter (1976) confirming the high uptake of estramustine in the rat ventral prostate after a single intravenous dose of estramustine phosphate, also found that after administration

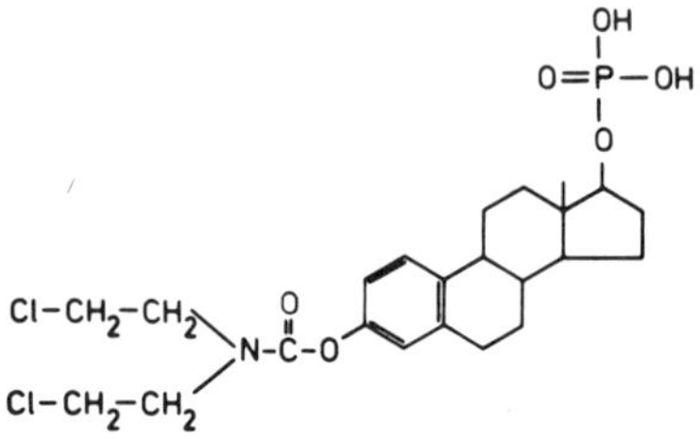

estramustine phosphate, Leo 299

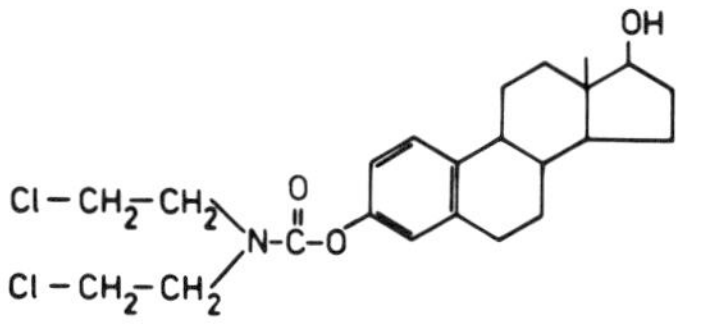

estramustine, Leo 275

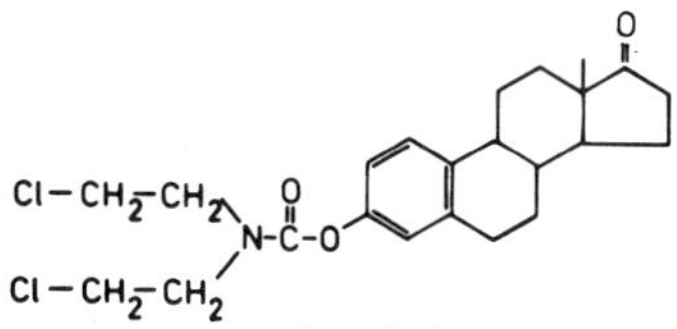

Leo 271

Fig. 1: Chemical formulae of estramustine phosphate (Leo 299), estramustine (Leo 275), and 17-dehydrogenated estramustine (Leo 271).

of the drug for three days (100 mg/kg body weight) the 17-dehydrogenated congener of estramustine, the estrone nitrogen mustard complex (Fig. 1), was accumulated in the ventral prostate.

These initial findings led to detailed studies on the mechanism(s) behind this uptake of estramustine phosphate metabolites, in the rat ventral prostate. Bearing in mind the possible existence of a receptor or receptor-like mechanism we wanted to use a labeled ligand of high specific activity in order to work at ligand levels comparable to those used in steroid receptor studies. Technical reasons (the phosphorylation step) prevented the synthesis of estramustine phosphate of the desired specific activity. Estramustine, however, tritiated in the estradiol moiety could be synthesized with high specific activity (80-110 Ci/mmole). Distribution studies in rats using this compound (0.8 μg/kg body weight) confirmed the earlier findings and also showed a time dependent concentration of radioactivity in the rat ventral prostate that did not occur in most other tissues (Forsgren *et al.*, 1979 & 1977). In contrast, radioactivity initially taken up by the ventral prostate after administration of

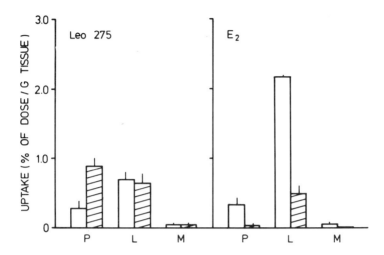

Fig. 2: Distribution of [^{3}H] estramustine (Leo 275) and [^{3}H] estradiol-17β (E$_2$) in rat ventral prostate (P), liver (L) and skeletal muscle (M). The results are expressed as a percentage of dose ± S.E. (n = 5) per g tissue wet weight 30 min. (white columns) and 2 hr (shadowed columns) after administration of 0.44 nmole [^{3}H] estramustine or 0.47 nmole [^{3}H] estradiol-17β to orchiectomized rats.

tritiated estradiol-17β (0.5 μg/kg body weight) rapidly vanished from the gland (Fig. 2). Simultaneous autoradiographic studies showed a continuous transport of radioactivity after administration of [^{3}H] estramustine through the epithelial cells into the secretory contents of the prostatic lumina (Appelgren *et al.*, 1978). This secretion of radioactivity did not take place after administration of [^{3}H] testosterone or [^{3}H] estradiol-17β.

Cytosol (105,000 x g supernatant) prepared from the rat ventral prostate gland obtained 2 hr after administration of [^{3}H] estramustine was separated by gel chromatography (Forsgren *et al.*, 1979). A major peak of radioactivity was eluted together with the main UV-absorbing peak. Thin-layer chromatography analysis of the radioactive material that was easily extracted from the eluate using organic solvent showed that it consisted mainly of estramustine.

The binding of estramustine by the rat ventral prostate was further studied *in vitro* using cytosol preparations (Forsgren *et al.*, 1979 , 1977 & 1978). Estramustine was bound to a much higher extent (Fig. 3) and to other macromolecular species (Fig. 4) than estradiol-17β or 5α-dihydrotestosterone. The *in vitro* binding of estramustine by rat ventral prostate cytosol occurred with a broad pH optimum between pH 7 and 8.5 with a maximum binding at pH 7.8. The

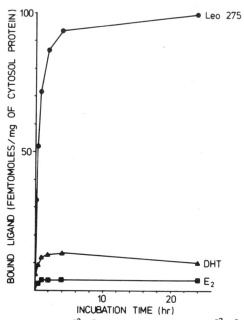

Fig. 3: Macromolecule-bound [³H] estramustine (●), 5α-[³H] dihydrotestoste-rone (▲), and [³H] estradiol-17β (■) after filtration on Sephadex G-25 of rat ventral prostate cytosol (11-13 mg of protein per ml) incubated at 0-4° C for various times with 1.2, 1.3 and 0.6 nmoles/l of the respective ligands, correspon-ding to 111, 104 and 45 fmoles of ligand per mg of protein. Each value is the mean of two determinations.

protein nature of the estramustine-binding species was showed by its insensitivity to DNase or RNase treatment. The estramustine-binding protein (EMBP) concentrated at pH 5 during isoelectric focusing in a sucrose gradient. Sucrose density gradient centrifugation at low ionic strength indicated a sedimentation coefficient of 3.7 S. Using this value and a Stokes radius of 2.9 nm (obtained by gel chromatography on a calibrated column) the molecular weight of EMBP was calcula-ted (Siegel *et al.*, 1966) to 44,000. Using the linear relationship be-tween the ratio of elution volume to void volume and the logarithm of the molecular weight (Determann *et al.*, 1966), this parameter was determined to 48,000 - 50,000.

Scatchard analysis (1949) of the binding characteristics of EMBP after incubation of rat ventral prostate cytosol with [³H] estramusti-ne at 15° C, yielded an apparent dissociation constant (K_d) of 10-30 nM (mean value 16.6 ± 2.6 (S.E.), n = 7) and a calculated maximal binding capacity of about 5 nmoles/mg total cytosol protein (mean value 4.6 ± 0.2 (S.E.), n = 7) (Fig. 5). The rate of

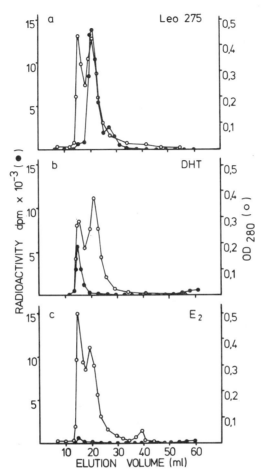

Fig. 4: Ultrogel AcA-54 chromatography of the macromolecular fraction obtained after Sephadex G-25 filtration of rat ventral prostate cytosol incubated for 4 hr at 0-4°C with a) [³H] estramustine (1.2 nM), b) 5α- [³H] dihydrotestosterone (1.4 nM), and c) [³H] estradiol-17β (2.0 nM). Protein concentrations were 13 mg (a, b) and 16 mg (c) per ml of cytosol. Absorbance at 280 nm (○); radioactivity (●).

dissociation of the estramustineprotein complex increased rapidly with temperature with half-lives of about 210, 80, 9 and 4 min. at 15°C, 22°C, 30°C, and 37°C, respectively. At 0°C no dissociation was found even after 24 hr. Since the dissociation rates were high compared to the degradation rates (see below), no corrections were made for the latter. The estramustinebinding protein in rat ventral prostate cytosol showed no sign of degradation after 24 hr at 0°C,

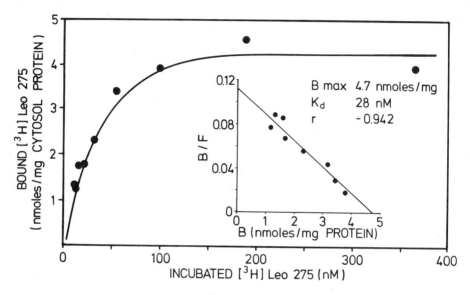

Fig. 5: Saturation and Scatchard analysis of binding of Leo 275 to rat ventral prostate cytosol. Each point represents the mean of duplicate samples. The Scatchard plot shows the specific binding after correction according to Chamness and McGuire (1975). Maximal specific binding was 4.7 nmoles/mg total cytosol protein (1.6 μg cytosol protein/ml incubate) with an apparent K_d of 28 nM (r = -0.942).

and degraded with half-lives of about 80, 30, 6, and 1.5 hr at 15°C, 22°C, 30°C, and 37°C, respectively (Forsgren *et al.,* 1979).

The ligand specificity of EMBP was examined using 10 nM [^{3}H] estramustine and various unlabeled steroids, steroid conjugates, and steroid nitrogen mustard derivatives in concentrations ranging from 1 nM to 45 μM. The result was expressed as a percentage of the amount of radioactivity bound in the absence of unlabeled competitor and plotted after logit transformation against the logarithm of the ratio between unlabeled competitor and labeled marker according to Rodbard *et al.,* (1968). None of the steroids or steroid conjugates inhibited the binding of [^{3}H] estramustine by more than 35% even at 45 μM concentration. The most efficient steroidal inhibitor at this concentration (4,500-fold excess versus the tracer) was progesterone (35% inhibition) followed by estrone (30%), pregnenolone (25%), androstenedione (20%), and dehydroepiandrosterone (10%). All the other steroids or steroid conjugates tested decreased the binding of the tracer by less than 10% when added in 4,500-fold excess (Table I). Those steroids and steroid conjugates were: estradiol-17β, 5α-dihydrotestosterone, testosterone, 19-nortestosterone,

5α-androstane-3β, 17β-diol, corticosterone, cortisol, dexamethasone, ethinylestradiol, estriol, diethylstilbestrol, estrone sulfate, estradiol-17β-3-sulfate, estradiol-17β-3, 17-disulfate, estrone glucuronide, and estradiol-17β-17-glucuronide.

TABLE I

Effect of various steroids and steroid conjugates on the binding of [^{3}H] estramustine by rat ventral prostate cytosol

Competitor (45 μM)	Bound ^{3}H Leo 275 (in % of control)
No competitor	100
Progesterone	65
Estrone	70
Pregnenolone	75
Androstenedione	80
Dehydroepiandrosterone	90
Other steroids or steroid conj.	> 90

Cytosol samples (200 μl, 1.6 μg protein/ml) were incubated at 15°C for 18 hr with 10 nM [^{3}H] estramustine in the presence of varying amounts (1 nM - 45 μM) of unlabeled steroids or steroid conjugates. After a treatment with dextran-coated charcoal the protein-bound radioactivity in the presence of competitor was expressed as a percentage of the radioactivity bound in the absence of competitor. The table shows the cytosol-binding of [^{3}H] estramustine ([^{3}H] Leo 275) in the presence of 45 μM competitor, i.e. a 4,500-fold excess of competitor relative to the concentration of the tracer. Estramustine gave 50% inhibition at two-fold excess.

In contrast, several of the nitrogen mustard derivatives tested gave rise to displacement curves with concentrations for 50% inhibition ranging from 15-25 nM to 6-8 μM, i.e. from two-fold to 700-fold excess of the unlabeled competitor versus the tracer. Comparison between the different concentrations required for 50% inhibition of [^{3}H] estramustine binding was only made for curves "parallel,, to the standard (estramustine) curve. A displacement curve was considered parallel to the standard curve when $p > 0.05$ when tested on the assumption on non-parallelism. "Parallelism" was considered to represent competitive inhibition of [^{3}H] estramustine binding, and "non-parallelism" ($p < 0.05$) was interpreted as the presence of different binding sites on the protein for the competing compound and estramustine and/or that the displacing effect was caused by factors other than pure competition for the estramustine-binding site. These concepts are illustrated in Fig. 6.

The effectiveness of the various competitors to inhibit the binding of [^{3}H] estramustine was calculated as "relative binding affinity"

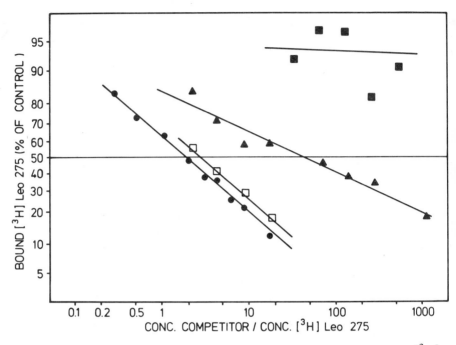

Fig. 6: Competition of some steroid mustard derivatives for binding of [³H] estramustine in rat ventral prostate cytosol. The resulting inhibitory curves are linearized by plotting logit Y versus log X, where Y = the ratio between the amount of [³H] Leo 275 bound in the presence and the absence of unlabeled competitor, and X = the ratio between concentration of unlabeled competitor and concentration of [³H] Leo 275 incubated, respectively. Each point represents the mean of duplicate samples. ●—●, estramustine (Leo 275); □—□, estramustine 17β-acetate (Leo 289); ▲—▲, estramustine 17β-propionate (Leo 358); ■—■, estramustine 17β-trimethylacetate (Leo 470). The curve of Leo 289 is "parallel" to that of Leo 275, the curves of Leo 358 and 470 are not owing to bulky substituents at position 17.

(RBA), expressed as the ratio of excess of estramustine required for 50% inhibition to excess of competitor required for 50% inhibition. Table II shows RBA of those steroid nitrogen mustard derivatives the displacement curves of which were "parallel" to the estramustine standard curve. Among the compounds tested but not listed in Table II (owing to "non-parallelism") were estramustine 17β-propionate (Leo 358), estramustine 17β-trimethylacetate (Leo 470), estramustine 17β-trimethylacetate (Leo 470), estramustine 17β-N-bis(2-chloroethyl)carbamate (Leo 453), estradiol-17β 17β-N-bis(2-chloroethyl)carbamate (Leo 298). 5α-dihydrotestosterone 17β-N-bis(2-chloroethyl)carbamate (Leo 543), and others. Leo 298, Leo 453, and Leo 543 gave similar "displacement curves" as Leo 470 (cf. Fig. 6).

TABLE II

	Leo no.	RBA		Leo no.	RBA
$R = -\overset{\overset{O}{\parallel}}{C}-N-(CH_2CH_2Cl)_2$			(structure, RO)	Leo 452	0.23
(structure, RO)	Leo 271	1.16	(structure, OH, RO)	Leo 524	0.16
(structure, OH, RO)	Leo 275	1.00	(structure, OH, --OOCCH₃, RO)	Leo 2035	0.02
(structure, H --OH, RO)	Leo 2179	1.00	(structure, OH, --OH, RO)	Leo 1611	0.01
(structure, OOCCH₃, RO)	Leo 289	0.77	(structure, O, RO, H)	Leo 451	0.007
(structure, OH, --C≡CH, RO)	Leo 675	0.44	(structure, OPO(OH)₂, RO)	Leo 299	0.002

Relative binding affinity (RBA) of some estrogen and non-estrogen nitrogen mustard derivatives for the estramustinebinding protein in the rat ventral prostate. Cytosol samples (200 μl, 1.6 μg protein/ml) were incubated at 15°C for 18 hr with 10 nM [³H] estramustine in the presence of varying amounts (1 nM - 45 μM) of unlabeled competitors. Bound radioactivity was analyzed by use of a dextran-coated charcoal technique and expressed as a percentage of the radioactivity bound in the absence of competitor. Under the experimental conditions used the concentration of unlabeled estramustine required for 50% inhibition was 20 nM, i.e. 2-fold excess, and saturation of the estramustine binding sites was accomplished at approximately 100 nM estramustine (cf. Fig. 5).

The results of the studies on the ligand specificity of EMBP showed that certain structural requirements are indispensable for "parallelism" and/or for efficient inhibition of estramustine binding. The natural steroids are very poor inhibitors of estramustine binding

(Table I). This does not necessarily mean, however, that the steroids do not bind at all to the binding sites of estramustine. It might just be that the binding affinity of the steroids is too low compared to that of estramustine to allow efficient competition. In order to exert efficient inhibition of the binding of estramustine the competitor evidently must be structurally similar to estramustine, i.e. the steroidal carrier must have the nitrogen mustard group attached at position 3 and bulky substituents at position 17 are not allowed (no derivatives with the nitrogen mustard attached to positions other than 3 and/or 17β have been available for testing). Furthermore, it seems that for the most efficient competition the carrier molecule must be of the estran series, since changing the benzene structure of the A-ring into a 5,6-double bond (the nitrogen mustard derivative of dehydroepiandrosterone, Leo 452, and androst-5-ene-3β,17β-diol, Leo 524, respectively) decreases the competitive capacity versus that of the corresponding estrogen derivatives by a factor of 5-6 (Table II). A still more decreased inhibitory effect is obtained with the nitrogen mustard derivative of the completely saturated carrier androsterone (3α-hydroxy-5α-androstan-17-one), Leo 451. However, it is not possible to make a relevant comparison between Leo 451 and Leo 524 because in Leo 451 the nitrogen mustard is attached perpendicularly (axial α-configuration) to the general plane of the A-ring of the carrier, while in Leo 524 the corresponding substituent lies in the plane (equatorial β-configuration). Thus, the most efficient inhibitors of estramustine binding among the compounds tested were those where the nitrogen mustard was attached to the phenolic hydroxy group of an estran carrier. Estrone, estradiol-17β, and estradiol-17α were the most suitable carriers. Bulky substituents at the 17-position of the estrogen moiety abolished the ability of the compound to competitively inhibit the binding of estramustine. However, already small substituents as in Leo 289 and Leo 675 (Table II) affected the inhibitory capacity. Substitution at the 16α-position of estramustine practically abolished the inhibitory effect although the small remaining effect was competitive.

Referring to the title of the Workshop, "The Use of Estrogens as Carriers of Cytotoxic Agents in Hormone Receptive Tumors" it might be relevant to mention that the estramustine-binding protein (EMBP), detected in the rat ventral prostate, is found also in other androgen-dependent tissues. Using a radioimmunoassay based on antibodies produced in rabbits against purified rat ventral prostate EMBP, cytosol preparations of various rat tissues were examined for their content of EMBP (Forsgren et al., 1979). In male rats EMBP was present in high levels in the ventral prostate (18-20% of the total cytosol protein content) and in lower amounts in the lateral and dorsal lobes of the prostate (0.8 and 0.2% of total cytosol protein, respectively). In addition, EMBP was found in lower amounts in other androgen-dependent tissues of the male rat (Table III).

TABLE III

Concentration of estramustine-binding protein in cytosol preparations from various tissues

Tissue	ng/mg of total cytosol protein	
	Male	Female
Ventral prostate	177,000 +	
Lateral prostate	8,350 +	
Dorsal prostate	1,817 +	
Coagulating gland	503 +	
Seminal vesicle	394 +	
Submaxillary gland	278 +	6 +
Adrenal gland	210 +	n.d. −
Preputial gland	184 +	n.d. −
Pancreas	167 −	167 −
Pituitary gland	63 +	n.d. −
Epididymis	50 +	
Thyroid gland	48 +	n.d. −
Cerebral cortex	28 +	99 +

Within-assay variation was ± 5.8% in samples ranging from 98 to 300 ng/ml (X = 166.3 ng/ml, n = 14), ± 12.2% in samples ranging from 50 to 116 ng/ml (X = 74.6 ng/ml, n = 11), and 16.1% in samples ranging from 11 to 56 ng/ml (X = 31.1 ng/ml, n = 14). Between-assay variation calculated as SD for a sample containing 75.5 ng/ml analyzed in six different assays was 10.8%. The least detectable dose (Feldman *et al.*, 1971) was 2.5 ng/ml. Values below 2.5 ng/ml are indicated by n.d. Tissues giving dose response curves of shape similar to those for ventral prostate are indicated by +; those giving curves of other shapes are indicated by −.

In male rats no EMBP was detected in the epiphysis, lung, liver, kidney, spleen, testis, skeletal muscle, or plasma. In female rats no EMBP was found in the epiphysis, pituitary gland, thyroid gland, lung, liver, adrenal gland, uterus, ovary, oviduct, vagina, preputial gland, skeletal muscle, or plasma, and in very small amounts in the kidney and spleen (4 and 3 ng/mg of total cytosol protein, respectively, with dose-response curves indicated by +).

The androgen dependency of EMBP has recently been studied in rat ventral prostate using the radioimmunoassay (Pousette *et al.*). Being rather low before puberty the EMBP concentration increases significantly at puberty. After orchiectomy of mature rats the amount of

EMBP decreases, while androgen treatment restores the concentration. Estrogen treatment of male rats decreases the EMBP content of the ventral prostate.

Recently, studies have been initiated to investigate the possible occurrence of EMBP or a similar protein in human prostate tissue. Scatchard analysis of binding data obtained for estramustine in cytosol from a specimen of benign prostatic hyperplasia (BPH) indicated the existence of a binding agent with the same affinity for estramustine (K_d = 35 nM) as that of rat EMBP. Gel filtration of the cytosol fraction of a BPH specimen revealed an estramustine binding macromolecule with a molecular weight of approximately 50,000. By sucrose gradient centrifugation of [^{3}H] estramustine-labeled cytosol two radioactive peaks were obtained at 3.2 S and 4.6 S, respectively. Following isoelectric focusing of a similar sample radioactivity was concentrated at pH 5. Finally, radioimmunoassay of serial dilution of cytosols from BPH tissue species gave dose-response curves identical to the standard curve for rat EMBP. It would therefore seem as if human prostate tissue contains a protein similar or identical to rat EMBP. Experiments are now in progress to investigate the nature of the estramustine-binding agent in the human prostate. Its possible presence in human prostate tissue may provide an explanation for the efficiency of estramustine phosphate in the treatment of prostatic carcinoma. Recent results of studies on the metabolism of estramustine phosphate in patients treated for long time with the drug show that high amounts of estramustine, Leo 275, and its 17-dehydrogenated congener, Leo 271, (10-50 and 100-500 ng/ml plasma, respectively) circulate in patients who receive 560-840 mg estramustine phosphate daily for several months (Gunnarsson et al., 1978). An estramustine- (and Leo 271-) binding agent in the human prostate may concentrate these compounds from the blood and provide the tissue with a high concentration of estrogen-nornitrogen mustard complexes, the exact mechanism of action of which within the prostatic cell remains to be explained. Sandberg and collaborators, intensively studying the metabolism of estramustine phosphate in man (for references, see Sandberg, 1980), have found that organ cultures of human normal, benign hyperplastic, or neoplastic prostatic tissue, in addition to the ability to take up estramustine phosphate, also had the capacity to dephosphorylate and hydrolyze the drug giving rise to estramustine, 17-dehydrogenated estramustine, free estrogens (estrogen-17β and estrone) and to liberation of the nornitrogen mustard carbamate moiety, the metabolic fate of which is still not elucidated. Thus, an estramustine-binding agent in the neoplastic tissue may provide the tissue with high amounts of these various metabolites of estramustine phosphate, and interindividual differences in tissue content of this agent might be related to varying responses in prostatic cancer patients treated with estramustine phosphate.

Further studies on the ligand specificity of this androgen dependent, estramustine-binding protein are now in progress to examine the possibility of linking anti-tumor agents other than nornitrogen mustard to a suitable carrier in order to improve the anti-tumor effectiveness in androgen dependent neoplastic tissue.

References

Appelgren, L.-E., Forsgren, B., Gustafsson, J.-A., Pousette, A., and Högberg, B. (1978). *Acta Pharmacol. Toxicol.* **43**, 368.

Chamness, G. C., and McGuire, W. L. (1975). *Steroids* **26**, 538.

Determann, H., and Michel, W. (1966). *J. Chromatogr.* **25**, 303.

Feldman, H., and Rodbard, D. (1971). In *"Principles of Competitive Protein Binding"* (W. D. Odell and W. H. Daughaday, eds.), p. 158, Lippincott, Philadelphia.

Forsgren, B., Björk, P., Carlström, K., Gustafsson, J.-A., Pousette, A., and Högberg, B. (1979). *Proc. Natl. Acad. Sci. (USA)* **76**, 3149.

Forsgren, B., Gustafsson, J.-A., Pousette, A., Högberg, B. (1979). *Cancer Res.* (in press).

Forsgren, B., and Högberg, B. (1977). In *"Research on Steroids"* (A. Vermeulen, P. Jungblut, A. Klopper, L. Lerner, and F. Sciarra, eds.). Vol. 7, p. 431. North-Holland Publishing Company, Amsterdam.

Forsgren, B., Högberg, B., Gustafsson, J.-A., and Pousette, A. (1978). *Acta. Pharm. Succ.* **15**, 23.

Gunnarsson, P. O., Nilsson, T., and Plym Forshell, G. (1978). *Urol. Res.* (submitted for publication).

Høisaeter, P. A. (1976). *Acta Endocrinol.* (Copenhagen) **82**, 661.

Jönsson, G., Högberg, B., and Nilsson, T. (1977). *Scand. J. Urol. Nephrol.* **11**, 231.

Könyves, T., and Liljekvist, J. (1976). In *"Biological Characterization of Human Tumours. Proceedings of the Sixth International Symposium on the Characterization of Human Tumours, Copenhagen, May 13-16, 1975"*. (Excerpta Medica International Congress Series No. 375). p. 98. Excerpta Medica, Amsterdam.

Plym Forshell, G., and Nilsson, H. (1974). *Acta Pharmacol. Toxicol.* **35** (Suppl. I), 28. (Abstract).

Pousette, A., Björk, P., Carlström, K., Forsgren, B., Högberg, B., and Gustafsson, J.-A. In preparation.

Rodbard, D., Rayford, P. L., Cooper, J. A., and Ross, G. T. (1968). *J. Clin. Endocrinol. Metab.* **28**, 1412.

Sandberg, A. A. (1980). This refers to the lecture by Dr. Sandberg at the present Workshop.

Scatchard, G. (1949). *Ann. N. Y. Acad. Sci.* **51**, 660.

Siegel, L. M., and Monty, K. J. (1966). *Biochem. Biophys. Acta* **112**, 346.

Discussion

Wittliff: It seems that the protein Dr. Forsgren has been talking about is the same as the one described by Dr. Heyns but I leave it to Dr. Heyns to discuss that.

Heyns: As already mentioned by Dr. Forsgren (1979) the "estramustine binding protein" described by his group is most probably identical to the "prostatic binding protein (PBP)", which we have been studying the last few years (Heyns and De Moor, 1977; Heyns et al., 1978). Indeed, both proteins are major components of rat prostatic secretion and show an identical amino acid composition. Furthermore, they share a number of other properties, such as size, subunit composition and isoelectric point. The "prostatein" described by Lea et al., (1979) also may be identical, although the reported properties do not fit as closely. Finally, the non-specific or α-protein binding of androgens in prostatic cytosol (Fang and Liao, 1971) and the "receptor" binding of pregnenolone (Karsznia et al., 1969) may be due to this protein. A detailed discussion of the physicochemical properties of this binding protein does not fit within the scope of this Workshop, but I would like to draw your attention to one physiological aspect, which may be of some importance: the hormonal regulation of this protein (Heyns et al., 1978b).

As shown in the figure, prostatic binding protein is strongly androgendependent. After castration there is a marked drop of its concentration, which returns to normal after androgen treatment. Estrogens do not produce a similar stimulation, but in intact animals they will

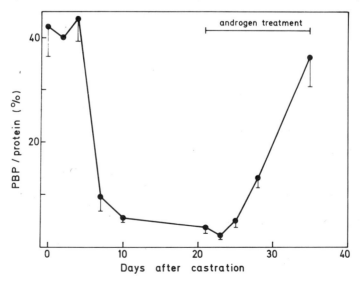

suppress the levels of androgens and consequently the levels of PBP. Since estramustine (Phosphate) is not devoid of estrogenic activity, one might expect that prolonged administration of this drug will reduce the level of the binding protein and thus impair the specific uptake mechanism. At this moment one can only speculate whether a similar phenomenon will occur in the normal human prostate or in prostatic tumors.

Sandberg: The protein described by Dr. Heyns has been described as a prostatic binding protein and the one described by Dr. Forsgren as estracyt binding protein. I think they both are the same as prostatine and the protein that Liao calls α-protein. They are all isolated from the same source and they all have the same characteristics. There are several features that are extremely interesting. It is a secretory protein and I think that Liao has found that there is a very strong binding of spermidine to this protein. We have identified a similar protein in human materials. Dr. Forsgren probably has data on that.

Forsgren: On a cytosol preparation of human benign prostatic hyperplasia labeled with tritiated estramustine we observe, on gel chromatography, that the MW of the binding macromolecule is about 50,000. We have not yet any data on the MW of the human as we have for the rat. Furthermore the complex was concentrated at the same pH in isoelectric focusing and it also sediments at 3.2 S and 4.6 S. We have now samples of what we call normal prostate. We have samples from the dorsal, lateral and median lobes of the human prostate and also samples of benign hyperplasia. The results of these experiments were ready last week, so I have no slides but I can tell you that we have a rather good binding of estramustine, at 3.7 S, in the cytosol of the dorsal lobe. We found approximately the same dissociation constant as in the rat but we have a rather low concentration of binding sites in the hyperplastic tissue. We have tried to make a radioimmunoassay for different samples of benign hyperplastic tissue. We observe large variations in the contents of something that cross reacts immunologically with our antibodies (against rat protein). However we don't know whether it is the same binding agent or something else. We are further looking into that.

Heuson: Do you have any idea what type of protein or enzyme this might be. Since apparently this binding is intracellular and since it is a secretory protein? Could it for example be acid phosphatase?

Forsgren: We don't have any idea right now.

Heyns: The important concentration of this binding protein in the rat ventral prostate suggests indeed, that it may correspond to a known functional component of this gland, showing by accident some steroid or estramustine binding. We have looked for phosphatase activity, but our results were negative.

Wittliff: Obviously, the human and the rat have not made a protein just to bind estramustine, Dr. Heyns, do you have any idea of its physiological function? Anything related to spermine or spermidine?

Heyns: I think that the spermidine binding protein is a different protein.

Harper: Dr. Heyns, according to the data presented by Dr. Forsgren there is a difference in the binding of androgen between his and yours.

Heyns: The apparent difference in specificity is due to the different affinity of the binding protein for the labeled steroid, which is used in the competition assay. Indeed, the affinity of estramustine is about a thousand times higher than the affinity for natural steroids, such as pregnenelone or androstenedione. For this reason the competition by these natural steroids is difficult to detect using (3H) estramustine, but shows up clearly, when (3H) pregnenelone of (3H) androstenedione are used for the measurement of binding.

Katzenellenbogen: It is amazing to see that estramustine is concentrated in the prostate. But if this is a cytosolic or secretory protein, perhaps it is preventing estramustine from entering the nucleus?

Wittliff: Yes, also in most biological systems, we see high affinity binders with low capacity. Here we have a protein that has a relatively high affinity and yet it represents 18% of the protein in the prostate. The protein is nearly purified and I am curious what its biological role is. Could you clarify how a protein with such a high affinity could come to such high concentrations.

Sandberg: You should not consider a secretory protein as an intercellular protein. When you homogenize the prostate, the secretion is in it and this is exactly where this binder is. So don't think that this binder represents 18% of the intracellular protein.

Heyns: Prostatic binding protein or estramustine binding protein is, indeed, a secretory protein. Due to homogenization, the protein in the acini and also in the secretory granules will be included in the "cytosol" fraction, resulting in a high "cytosolic" concentration. The concentration in the cytoplasm, however, is probably very low. With regard to your question on the spermine-or spermidine-binding protein described by Liao, this protein shows markedly different physiochemical properties, although I cannot completely rule out the possibility that it corresponds to a subunit or peptide component of prostatic binding protein.

References

Fang, S. and Liao, S., 1971. Androgen receptors. Steroid and tissue specific retention of 17-β-hydroxy-5α-androstane-3-one by the cell nuclei of the ventral prostate. *J. Biol. Chem,* **246**, 16-24.

Forsgren, B., Björk P., Carlström, K. Gustafsson, J. A., Pousette, A. and Högberg B., 1979. Purification and distribution of a major protein mustard derivative of estradiol-17β. *Prod. Nat. Acad. Sci.,* **76**, 3149-3153.

Heyns, W., and De Moor, P., 1977. Prostate binding protein: a steroid binding secreted by rat prostate. *Eur. J. Biochem.,* **78**, 921-220.

Heyns, W., Peeters, A., Moris, J., Rombouts, W. and De Moor, P., 1978. Purification and characterisation of prostatic binding protein and its subunits. *Eur. J. Biochem.,* **89**, 181-186.

Heyns, W., Van Damme, B. and De Moor, P., 1978. Secretion of prostatic binding protein by rat ventral prostate. Influence of age and androgen. *Endocrinology,* **89**, 1090-1095.

Karsznia, R., Wyss, R. H., Leroy Heinrichs, W. M. and Herrmann, W. I., 1969. Binding of pregnenolone and progesterone by prostatic "receptor" proteins. *Endocrinology,* **84**, 1238-1246.

Lea, O. A., Petiwsz, P. and French, F. S., 1979. Prostatein: a major secretory protein of the rat ventral prostate., *J. Biol. Chem.,* **254**, 6196-6202.

PROSPECTS FOR COMPOUNDS UTILIZING ESTROGENS AS CARRIERS OF CYTOTOXIC MOLECULES IN CANCER TREATMENT

RAPHAEL CATANE, SALVADOR BRUNO, FRANCO M. MUGGIA

Cancer Therapy Evaluation Program, Division of Cancer Treatment, National Cancer Institute, Bethesda, Maryland 20205, U.S.A.

Introduction

Even before the identification of hormone receptors, chemists had explored the use of hormones as carriers for cytotoxic agents. Their introduction into clinical trial was met with variable success, and interest in studying these compounds temporarily declined. More recently, there has been a renewal of interest based on our expanded ability to study mechanisms of hormone action and effects on hormone-dependent tumor cell lines. Such studies will be required to demonstrate advantages over cytotoxic drugs and hormones given independently (Von Hoff *et al.*, 1977). Two alkylating agents with an estrogen backbone have been studied in the U.S.A. Estradiol Mustard (NSC-112259) and Estramustine Phosphate (Estracyt) (NSC-89197) (Figures 1 and 2).

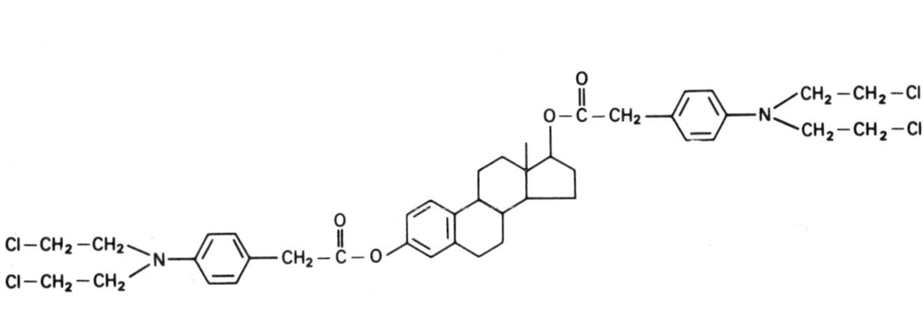

Fig. 1: Chemical structure of estradiol mustard.

Mechanism of Action of Cytotoxic Agents Linked to Estrogen Carriers

As indicated, our knowledge of these compounds has been largely empirical. Mechanisms of action can be studied through new techniques and the development of hypotheses may be helpful in explaining these experimentally. Two mechanisms may be involved in enhancing the antitumor selectivity of the cytotoxic-estrogen agents over that of a cytotoxic compound by itself: one is a facilitated transport of the active agent to the cellular targets and the second is enhanced activation of the cytotoxic molecule at the target. Both mechanisms may actually be operative in any one instance.

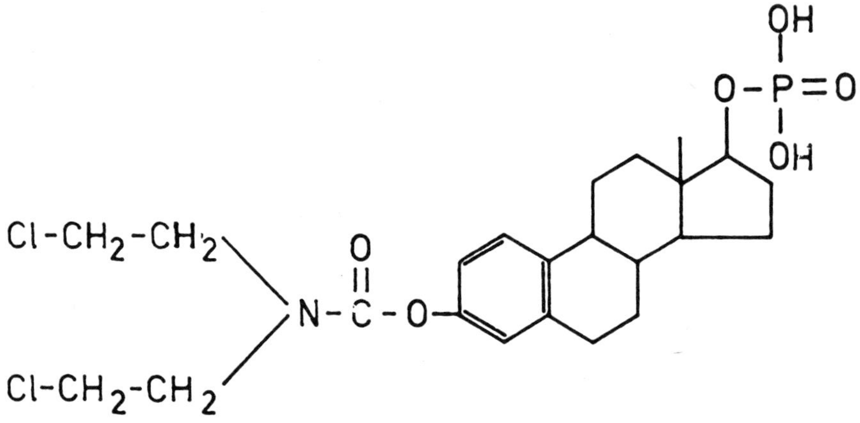

Fig. 2: Structural formula of estramustine phosphate (Estracyt).

For the carrier hypothesis to be implicated, the estrogen moiety of the molecule ought to be able to bind to an estrogen receptor (ER). For both Estradiol Mustard (EM) and Estramustine Phosphate (EMP), however, affinity to ER's, when measured, has been much lower than for estradiol (Everson et al., 1974; Wittliff et al., 1978). The dephosphorylation derivative of EMP was found to have higher affinity to ER than its parent compound (Leclercq et al., 1976). In vivo, EMP is rapidly dephosphorylated to estramustine (Tritsch, et al., 1974). This product must be considered in studying the action of the parent compound.

It is of interest that EMP has been reported to have some affinity for androgen receptors (Nilsson *et al.*, 1976), and it has also been suggested recently that a specific EMP-binding macromolecule "receptor" is present in the prostate (Forsgren *et al.*, 1978). EMP accumulates in areas presumably rich in this receptor (Appelgren *et al.*, 1978). The number of receptors available may, in fact, be subject to hormonal control. This phenomenon may account for the increased uptake of EMP by the prostate without increasing the uptake of estradiol following administration of testosterone to castrated mice (Catane, R., Sandberg, A. A., and Kirdani, R. Y., unpublished results).

The second mechanism for an enchanced antitumor action is selective activation of the molecule by the target tissue. Hydrolysis activates EMP, liberating the cytotoxic moiety; this was shown to be more readily accomplished by prostatic tissue than other tissues (Kadohama *et al.*, 1978). A chemically similar agent with prednisone as a carrier, prednimustine, is also activated by hydrolysis; in a detailed study, it was demonstrated that hydrolysis occurred preferentially in tumors, whereas the target organs at risk (especially the bone marrow) had only minimal hydrolytic activity (Wilkinson *et al.*, 1978).

Clinical Experience

Estradiol Mustard (EM) was introduced following antitumor activity demonstrable in various animal tumors (Vollmer *et al.*, 1973; Wittliff *et al.*, 1978). However, in the initial clinical trial including broad Phase II experience by the Eastern Cooperative Oncology Group, the response rate was very poor (Schapira *et al.*, 1978). Only one patient out of 17 with breast cancer had an objective response, and five other patients had subjective improvement while showing no progression. In a variety of other tumors, no responses were seen (Table I). Moreover, hematologic toxicity was prominent.

The initial pilot studies with estramustine phosphate (EMP) in the U.S.A. were performed at Roswell Park Memorial Institute and indicated promising activity in patients with prostatic cancer no longer responding to hormonal therapy (Table II). EMP alone gave an 18% objective response rate in those patients (Mittelman *et al.*, 1976). Subsequently, EMP was combined with prednimustine, another steroidalalkylating agent compound, and the resulting response rate was 24% (Catane *et al.*, 1977). When EMP was combined with methotrexate and cis-platinum, four out of nine patients responded, while none of the 21 patients treated with EMP and methyl-CCNU responded (Madajewicz *et al.*, 1979). These studies were encouraging because of

TABLE I
ECOG Study of Estradiol Mustard Activity*

Tumor	Partial Response	Stable	Progression	Total
Breast Cancer	1	5	11	17
Other Malignancies	0	8	14	22

* Pollow et al., 1978

durability of some responses (Catane et al., 1976), frequent sub-jective improvement, and good tolerance of the drug.

TABLE II
Objective Response Rate Obtained with Estramustine Phosphate (EMP) in
Patients with Advanced Hormone Resistant Prostatic Cancer;
the Roswell Park experience

Treatment	Objective Response Rate
EMP alone	8/44 (18 %)
EMP + Prednimustine	5/21 (24 %)
EMP + MeCCNU	0/21
EMP + Cis-Platinum + MTX	4/9

The National Prostatic Cancer Project in a randomized study indicated an advantage of EMP over "standard" therapy (Murphy et al., 1977), and they also confirmed the frequent improvement in subjective criteria (weight gain, improved performance status, pain relief and correction of anemia). Similar conclusions have been drawn in a study at the University of Wisconsin (Benson et al., 1979). However, in combination with other agents (Table III), conflicting results have been reported (Kennealey, et al., 1978; Murphy et al., 1979), underlining the inherently difficult assessment of response in this disease. The absence of easily measurable disease is compounded in this instance by the inaccuracies in defining estrogen resistance. Additional clinical studies, perhaps utilizing endpoints as time-to-treatment failure, are needed to shed further light on the value of EMP relative to other therapeutic measures. Moreover, the National Prostatic Cancer Project is studying EMP as a front line treatment.

In addition to studies in prostatic cancer, EMP has also been tried in malignant melanoma. There has been some preliminary indication of activity in patients who were refractory to DTIC chemotherapy (Didolkar et al., 1978). In view of this preliminary experience,

TABLE III
Estramustine Phosphate (EMP) in Prostatic Cancer

Treatment	Partial Response (%)		Stable	Progression	Total
EMP alone[a] (2)	5	(10)	30	16	51
EMP alone (19)[b]	3	(6.5)	11	32	46
EMP and Predni-mustine (13)[b]	1	(2)	6	47	54
EMP and 5-Fluoro-uracil (20)[c]	3	(12)	8	14	25

[a] University of Wisconsin.
[b] National Prostatic Cancer Project.
[c] Yale University.

additional studies are also needed in conditions other than prostatic cancer (Von Hoff *et al.,* 1977).

Future Areas of Research

If the mechanism involved is related to selective affinity of these compounds for hormone receptors, the prospect for this group of compounds may be wider than appreciated. A number of tumors have been recently shown to possess estrogen receptors. In addition to breast cancer and endometrial carcinoma (Pollow *et al.,* 1978, Wittliff *et al.,* 1971), tumors like hypernephroma (Bojar *et al.,* 1976), melanoma (Fisher *et al.,* 1978), hepatocarcinoma (Monges *et al.,* 1977), prostatic carcinoma (Gustafsson *et al.,* 1978), ovarian adenocarcinoma (Holt *et al.,* 1979), and colon adenocarcinoma (McClendon *et al.,* 1977) have all been shown to have ERs. Clinical studies with this class of compounds should be considered in these areas.

Laboratory studies may also be helpful in further elucidating the antitumor selectivity of these compounds. The availability of human tumor cell lines with variable ER content and the ability to grow them in nude mice render such a system useful in correlating the antitumor activity of these compounds with ER content. Such suggestions arose from a recent workshop held by the Cancer Therapy Evaluation Program at the National Cancer Institute (Lippman *et al.,* 1978).

Conclusions

In summary, the future prospect of the cytotoxic agents–estrogen compounds depends on the following:

1. More insight into the prevalence of hormone receptors in human tumors and their importance in tumor biology.
2. Synthesis and study of agents which are selectively taken up by hormone receptors or which are activated by tumors, or both.
3. Well designed clinical studies supplemented if possible with laboratory determinations of indicators of hormonal responsiveness of individual tumors.

References

Appelgren, L. E., Forsgren, B., Gustafsson, J. A., Pousette, A., and Hugberg, B. (1978). *Acta Pharmacol. Toxicol.* **43**, 368.

Benson, R. C., Wear, J. B., and Gill, G. M. (1979). *J. Urol.* **121**, 452.

Bojar, H., Dreyfurst, R., Belzer, K., Staib, W., and Wittliff, J. L. (1976). *J. Clin. Chem. Clin. Biochem.* **14**, 521.

Catane, R., Kaufman, J., Mittelman, A., and Murphy, G. P. (1977). *J. Urol.* **117**, 332.

Catane, R., Mittelman, A., Kaufman, J., and Murphy, G. P. (1976). *N. Y. State J. Med.* **76**, 1978.

Didolkar, M. S., Catane, R., Lopez, R., and Holyoke, E. D. (1978). *Proc. Am. Assoc Cancer Res. Am. Soc. Clin. Oncol.* **19**, 381.

Everson, R. B., Turnell, R. W., Wittliff, J. L., and Hall, T. C. (1974). *Cancer Chemother. Rep.* **58**, 353.

Fisher, R. I., Neifeld, J. P., and Lippman, M. E. (1978). *Lancet* **2**, 337.

Forsgren, B., Hogberg, B., Gustafsson, J. A., and Pousette, A. (1978). *Acta Pharm. Suec.* **15**, 23.

Gustafsson, J. A., Ekman, P., Snochowski, M., Zetterberg, A., Pousette, A., and Hogberg, B. (1978). *Cancer Res.* **38**, 4345.

Holt, J. A., Caputo, T. A., Kelly, K. M., Greenwald, P., and Chorost, S. (1979). *Obstet. Gynecol.* **53**, 50.

Kadohama, N., Kirdani, R. Y., Murphy, G. P., and Sandberg, A. A. (1978). *J. Urol.* **119**, 235.

Kennealey, G. T., Marsh, J. C., Welch, D. A., Iamkis, M. D., and Gill, G. M. (1978). *Proc. Am. Assoc. Cancer Res. Am. Soc. Clin. Oncol.* **12**, 394.

Leclercq, G., Heuson, J. C., and Deboel, M. C. (1976). *Cancer Treat. Rep. Pharmacokin.* **2**, 77.

Lippman, M. E., Heuson, J. C., and Muggia, F. M. (1978). *Cancer Treat. Rep.* **62**, 1267.

Madajewicz, S., Catane, R., Mittelman, A., Wajsman, Z., and Murphy, G. P. (1979). *Oncology.* In press.

McClendon, J. E., Appleby, D., Claudon, D. B., Donegan, W. M., and DeCosse, J. J. (1977). *Arch. Surg.* **112**, 240.

Mittelman, A., Shukla, S. K., and Murphy, G. P. (1976). *J. Urol.* **115**, 409.

Monges, A., Treffot, M. H., Margin, P., Girodroux, C., and Rampol, M. (1977). *Gastroenterol. Clin. Biol.* **1**, 302.

Murphy, G. P., Gibbons, R. P., Johnson, D. E., Loening, S. A., Prout, G. R., Schmidt, J. D., J. D., Bross, D. S., Chu, T. M., Gaeta, J. F., Saroff, J., and Scott, W. W. (1977). *J. Urol.* **118**, 288.

Murphy, G. P., Gibbons, R. P., Johnson, D. E., Prout, G. R., Schmidt, J. D., Soloway, M. S., Loening, S. A., Chu, T. M., Gaeta, J. F., Saroff, J., Wajsman,

Z., Slack, N., and Scott, W. W. (1979). *J. Urol.* **121**, 763.

Nilsson, I., Liskowski, L., and Nilsson, T. (1976). *Urology* **8**, 118.

Pollow, K., Pollow, B., and Schmidt-Gollwitzer, M. (1978). *J. Mol. Med.* **3**, 71.

Schapira, D., Hall, T. C., Bennett, J. M., Lavin, P., Colsky, J., Perlia, C., Brodovsky, H., and Shnider, B. (1978). *Cancer Clin. Trial* **1**, 5.

Tritsch, G. L., Shukla, S. K., Mittelman, A., and Murphy, G. P. (1974). *Invest. Urol.* **12**, 38.

Vollmer, E. P., Taylor, D. J., Masnyk, I. J., Cooney, D., Levine, B., and Piczak, C. (1973). *Cancer Chemother. Rep.* **4**(3), 121.

Von Hoff, D. D., Rozencweig, M., Slavik, M., and Muggia, F. M. (1977). *J. Urol.* **117**, 464.

Wilkinson, R., Gunnarson, P. O., Plym-Furshell, G., Renshow, J., and Harrap, K. R. (1978). *Excerpta Med. Int. Congr. Ser.* **420**, 260.

Wittliff, J. L., Hilf, R., Brooks, W. F., Savlov, E. D., Hall, T. C., and Orlando, R. A. (1971). *Cancer. Res.* **32**, 1983.

Wittliff, J. L., Weidner, N., Everson, R. B. and Hall, T. C. (1978). *Cancer Treat. Rep.* **62**, 1262.

Wittliff, J. L., Weidner, N., Park, D. C., Everson, R. B., and Hall, T. C. (1978). *Cancer Treat. Rep.* **62**, 1260.

Discussion

Wittliff: Have you seen any evidence for the hypothesis that some compounds may require an enzymatic step intracellularly for activation?

Catane: There is an agent for which there are data in this direction. This is prednimustine, an agent similar to estracyt. Is consists of chlorambacil linked to prednisone and this compound is activated by hydrolysis. Moreover it was shown by Wilkinson that hydrolysis takes place better in tumors than in bone marrow. Since the toxicity of chlorambacil results in myelosuppression it was gratifying to see that the tumor hydrolyzes prednimustine better than the bone marrow. It was shown that the therapeutic index of the drug is better than just giving alkylating agents.

Paridaens: Dr. Catane, how long do you treat these patients?

Catane: This is a continuous treatment. We have patients who are actually treated for three to four years and they are doing well. Some patients just discontinued treatment by themselves and they are also doing well. This would mean that, in the future, we can stop with the treatment in patients who respond well after taking the drug for a year.

Heuson: Dr. Catane, I would like to know if this compound produces myelosuppression.

Catane: The toxicity is more on the gastrointestinal system. We give approximately one gram per day or one gram and a half per day. We cannot give more because of gastrointestinal problems like nausea and vomiting. At this dose you almost never get myelosuppression.

PANEL DISCUSSION

Hamacher: The number 15,000 of compounds that ICI is testing every year has impressed me. It seems that from a chemical point of view one has to look for a rational design. The first question is: on which position of the steroid should we put the cytotoxic group. The other question deals with the reactivity of the cytotoxic group. If you have cytotoxic groups that are too reactive, they will react too early. How reactive should a cytotoxic group be?

Catane: The alkylating part of the molecule was not really discussed. Most of the agents proposed here were just alkylating agents, except for a few like the Vinca alkaloids and the 5 FU; but what about all the other active agents we have today like platinum, bleomycine, actinomycin D etc. Maybe we should also think about those agents.

Wittliff: I do not think that we have any guidelines for the reactivity of the alkylating agents.

Könyves: I think that it is not possible to answer this because it depends on which position you put it on. It is not a mixture, it is one compound. Furthermore if you have a good alkylating agent directly linked to the steroid in the 11β position the reactivity will be different from the reactivity of a compound with an indirect link at the same position.

Wittliff: Yes, but don't you think that Dr. Catane's suggestion of adding other chemotherapeutic agents could really lead to some innovative chemistry?

Sandberg. We are going to be faced with that anyway, no single agent is going to cure breast cancer; we may have to use a battery of anti-estrogens and several chemotherapeutic agents. The sooner we get into that, the more compounds we will obtain and the more chances we will have to do something about breast cancer.

Katzenellenbogen: I think that there are many considerations; one of them is the accessibility and this is a point that Dr. Zeelen mentioned earlier. If the steroid is going to be bound to the receptor and not going to release the cytotoxic agent, it must fulfill certain requirements to reach DNA. The target of methotrexate is not DNA. This cytotoxic agent is going to be active while it is still under form of conjugate. I do not think that 5 FU is going to be active while it is attached to the estrogen. The situation becomes quite complex, one has to think about the activity of the conjugate versus the free compound and the accessibility of the target relative to the subcellular localization of the receptor.

Griffiths. But in relation to this, do we not assume that in some point in time the steroid comes off the receptor and is free in the nucleus?

Forsgren: But in that case you are back to the situation where you administer the compound, if you expect the complex to be active after coming off the receptor, it must be similarly active before it attaches on it.

Griffiths: Yes, but you are using the receptor to get it selectivily to the target organ.

Foster: Is it necessary to have translocation to the nucleus. If you have irreversible binding to the receptor, would that not be a successful way to be cytotoxic.

Sandberg: You would be using a cyanide for the receptor?

Griffiths: What is wrong with tamoxifen now? It works that same way. Tamoxifen does not inhibit translocation but impairs replenishment and as long as you are giving it, it inhibits receptor formation. Furthermore it is a non toxic agent.

Katzenellenbogen: Yes, but don't you have to take into consideration that the receptor is resynthesized?

Wittliff: Yes, but the receptor itself is important in the resynthesis of itself. Estradiol alone will not stimulate the receptor formation; it has to be bound to the receptor. So if you are damaging the receptor, you will not be replenishing it.

GENERAL DISCUSSION

Raus: I would like to ask a question to the panel on the screening of these compounds. I agree that due to the amount of material available, it is sometimes very difficult to start with *in vivo* screening but don't you think that it is a little bit dangerous to start with *in vitro* screening and make selections of the drugs based on this *in vitro* screening. I can imagine that there are compounds that will be active *in vitro* and that will not be active *in vivo* and vice versa.

Leclercq: That is true but if you have only 2 mg of the compound you have no other choice.

Wittliff: But what do you recommend, Dr. Leclercq? Would it be best to screen in tissue cultures cells because of the limited quantity of the material?

Leclercq: We believe that is the best, but because of the amount of material we usually start with binding studies *in vitro*.

Catane: If we don't have enough material and we have to do *in vitro* studies why should we not test the agents on tumor cell lines and also on normal cell lines like bone marrow. This would show some selectivity because an agent could be very active but also very toxic.

Könyves: Yes, when we look at the toxicity in breast tumor cells and at the toxicity in bone marrow, you will have quite a lot of information. You can determine the L50 in tumor cells and the L50 in bone marrow cells. This is a good preliminary screening. At least if you are talking of *in vitro* screening only.

Griffiths: Well, that is right. You cannot get large amounts of these materials, so you have to use cell lines.

Foster: I have a question related to the early stage of testing. Do you feel that metabolism of these compounds could be important? You can obtain some information on metabolism by using microsomal systems, especially since we are dealing with very small amounts of material. For some compounds metabolism might be important for others not. If one does this, one might get some guidelines on how to proceed further. I think that this relates to what Dr. Raus was asking on the *in vitro* versus the *in vivo* situation. Do you think that these metabolic studies could be useful?

Griffiths: You are thinking of making some metabolites in the event that some of these might work better than the original compounds?

Foster: Well, what I am thinking of is, if you do a simple microsomal metabolism and if you find a very extensive metabolism, then you ought to consider whether testing the compound per se is going to be particularly helpful. Some of the metabolites might have a different type of activity.

Wittliff: I think that we can propose the following scheme for *in vitro* screening:
1. Steroid binding *in vitro*
2. Microsomal metabolism of the compound
3. Effects on cell cultures (normal and neoplastic)
4. Stability in blood / biological fluid
5. Microbiological assay

How many of you on the panel feel studies of the drug's interaction with biological fluids, not microsomes, not extracts, but plasma and so on would be useful?

Katzenellenbogen: I think certainly any compound that is direct-acting should be tested in serum. There are nucleophiles that could rapidly be deactivated in some of these tissues.

Sandberg: I suggest to test the stability in whole blood, because pred-nimustine is hydrolyzed very quickly in the blood whereas estracyt is not. Since most of the compounds we have been discussing are conjugates. I think that it is very important to know whether they are hydrolyzed in the blood. I think you should also carry out "microbiological assays". Some of the chemotherapeutic agents were originally tested on enzyme systems of bacteria.

Könyves: Do you think that a combination of all these 5 items will give you the right answers. One tumor *in vivo* gives more information than a combination of these 5 points.

Wittliff: Do you mean that a combination of all 5 tests that I have written down here do not collectively give you the same quantity of information that you would get from one solid tumor experiment?

Sandberg: I thought that we were starting from the proposition that we had only 1 mg of material, if you have large amounts, of course.

Wittliff: But I think that even if you have a large amount of compound, Dr. Catane can describe this better, NIH has been testing thousands of compounds. I don't think that we can afford to do animal studies on all of these.

Catane: At the NIH, in the department of cancer treatment, they screen about 15,000 anticancer agents every year and only a few hundred pass the preliminary screening. A few hundred are tested in cell lines and about half of them have preliminary animal trials and that means a few hundred. Only 12 to 15 compounds a year are considered to be effective in animals. And of these 15 about 10 are tried in humans; the other five are dropped because of severe toxicity or unpredictable toxicity or pharmacological problems. Of these agents 1 or 2 compounds a year become marginally active and, as you know, the last ten or twelve years we have found only a few marginally active anticancer agents. So I think that these 5 steps are necessary and should be done: otherwise we would be wasting time and money by doing animal studies.

Wittliff: The studies that have originally been done with tamoxifen really provided the guiding principles what went on in the human trials. Dr. Griffiths do you agree with that?

Griffiths: Yes, but again ICI is making a lot of material. So you could do both *in vitro* and *in vivo* studies.

Katzenellenbogen: If you are just interested in developing any improved cytotoxic agent, then you should find out what you will be doing first but if you are really trying to design an agent that works by a receptor-mediated process, then I think you must draw special attention to step number 1. On the other hand if we had done that with estracyt, then we would have dropped it right away. The other thing is the amount of compound available, and there is probably a difference between the amount provided by pharmaceutical companies and academic chemists.

Wittliff: I would like to have a concensus about the estracyt association with the estrogen receptor *in vitro*. Dr. Forsgren, do you agree or do you have any evidence that it binds to the estrogen receptor?

Forsgren: I have carried out a gel chromatography of cytosol from the rat uterus labeled with radioactive estramustine. I will not say that it does not bind but I could not elute any radioactivity with the macromolecular fraction. So if it was bound to something in the uterine cytosol the binding affinity must have been very low. On the contrary when I used prostatic cytosol I got about 50% of the radioactivity bound to the proteins. In conclusion I would say that I have not succeeded in binding radioactive estramustine to a rat uterine cytosol.

Wittliff: What about you, Dr. Leclercq?

Leclercq: I tested estramustine some years ago and there was no significant binding of the drug. There was some kind of binding but this was probably due to the estrogen that is released by the hydrolysis of the drug.

Forsgren: I would like to make a comment on that. Dr. Leclercq used unlabeled estramustine phosphate to compete with labeled estradiol and when you do such experiments, you put in about 10,000 times the amount of the unlabeled compound versus the labeled compound. This means that if you have 0.01% impurities of unlabeled estradiol in your unlabeled estramustine phosphate, you have a relatively great amount of competitor. That is why we have used the labeled compound to avoid these problems. I would like to take the opportunity to say that, of course, the same reasoning applies to my competition experiments.

Wittliff: We repeated your experiments using the unlabeled estramustine phosphate and in uterus we found the same sort of results. When we used estrogen receptors from the lactating mammary gland we got an inhibition in the 8 S region. Again it may be due to some hydrolysate but when we did a radioimmunoassay we could not detect that amount of estradiol. We cannot agree whether it binds or not but I would like to indicate that in mammary cells it does bind to the receptor.

Forsgren: We have used double labeled estramustine phosphate, injected in a DMBA tumor bearing rat and there is radioactive uptake by the tumors. The ratio of 3H to C14 is approximately 1, which indicates that the molecule is intact. However we don't know whether it is bound to the receptor or to another protein that the tumor maybe secretes. We did an incubation of the DMBA cytosol with estramustine and we found binding in the void volume of the sephadex column which indicates that there is some binding to high molecular weight proteins.

Griffiths: Is there estramustine phosphate in the nucleus of the prostate? Does it go to the nucleus?

Forsgren: We have tried but we have only a few dpm's. I am not certain whether the intact molecule goes in the nucleus.

Wittliff: Maybe cell culture experiments can provide us with some information on the ability of the compound to be translocated while it is intact.

Blickenstaff: Assuming that one goes through these five steps followed by animal experiments, do you agree that the DMBA-induced mammary carcinoma is the first kind of animal to be tested?

Wittliff: Yes, that is an important question, what would be the best tumor animal model for estrogen-linked cytotoxic compounds?

Griffiths: We would consider the DMBA tumor because we know so much about it and once you have build a lot of background information, then of course it is the ideal experimental model.

Leclercq: I agree. Presently it is the DMBA tumor but as I have shown on my slides there is a new tumor transplanted in the mouse isolated by Medina.

We have it in our lab presently and this tumor is more easy to work with than an induced tumor. It regresses after ovariectomy and it regrows after estrogen administration, so it is an estrogen-dependent tumor, it has estradiol receptors like most DMBA mammary tumors and J. Clark in Houston has shown that when you inject estrogen into the animal the tumor develops progesterone receptors. It seems to be an excellent model.

Wittliff: It is called the MXP and that is in the mouse?

Leclercq: Yes, there is a paper by Watson Medina and Clark in Cancer Research in 1977. I believe that this would be a good model to use for the screening of these drugs.

Catane: It is our experience that no tumor model predicts what happens in the human. What we usually do is : we take a panel of tumors with several aspects and if a high number of tumors respond, then there is a better chance that it will work in the human. Recently human tumors transplanted in nude mice were used and we expect a lot from them although we do not really know whether they will be better than the usual tumors.

Wittliff: A problem with the nude mice is that only a few laboratories will be able to use nude mice because of the expenses.

Forsgren: Going back to the original question and the use of the DMBA tumors as a model. In spite of the fact that we observed an effect of estracyt on the DMBA tumor, the first clinical trials were negative. So it is not certain that you will get the right answer by using these animal models.

Griffiths: It is important to see whether the compound gets into the animal tumor and to see what its effect is. This is very relevant because ICI developed tamoxifen which is one of the best drugs developed in the last few years for cancer and we are still talking about which of the metabolites causes the effect on the tumor and it is already being used clinically. Tamoxifen was simply tested in the DMBA tumor, that means that for tamoxifen it was the right criterion.

SUBJECT INDEX